Philosophical Medical Ethics

Philosophical Medical Ethics

Raanan Gillon BA (philosophy) MB BS MRCP (UK)

Director, Imperial College Health Service
Editor, Journal of Medical Ethics
Deputy Director, Institute of Medical Ethics,
London, UK
Senior Fellow, Centre for Medical Law and Ethics,
Kings College, University of London

A Wiley Medical Publication
Published on behalf of
The British Medical Journal

JOHN WILEY & SONS
Chichester · New York · Brisbane · Toronto · Singapore

Library of Congress Cataloging-in-Publication Data:

Gillon, Raanan
  Philosophical medical ethics.

  (A Wiley medical publication)
  "Published on behalf of the British medical journal."
  Includes index.
  1. Medical ethics—Philosophy.   I. British medical
journal.   II. Title III. Series. [DNLM: 1. Ethics,
Medical.   2. Philosophy, Medical. W 50 G483p]
R725.5.G55   1986   174'.2   86—15749
ISBN 0 471 91222 0

British Library Cataloguing in Publication Data:

Gillon, Raanan
  Philosophical medical ethics.
  1. Medical ethics
  I. Title
174'.2   R724

ISBN 0 471 91222 0

Printed and bound in Great Britain by
Antony Rowe Ltd, Chippenham, Wiltshire

Contents

Preface

This book, originally written as a series of articles in the *British Medical Journal*, is aimed at any and all intelligent people who are interested in thinking critically about the many moral problems that arise in medical practice. It is written from my perspective as a philosophically trained practising general practitioner, perplexed by the moral problems that face me as a member of the medical profession and unwilling to rely merely on received wisdom. Doctors, it seems to me, tend to be rather reluctant to confront and think critically about medico-moral issues and three equally uncritical approaches are common: pontification, abstention and scepticism. The pontificators think they don't need critical medical ethics because, whether they are reactionary or radical, religious or atheistic, left wing or right wing, they *know* the answers. The abstainers—ours is not to reason why, ours is but to do and sigh—find it all too difficult. The sceptics think it is either impossible in principle, useless or irrelevant in practice, or a private matter for the individual and his conscience.

Each group—and these attitudes are by no means confined to members of the medical profession—will find its views challenged in this book. To the pontificators I recommend starting by reading the last chapter—you will almost certainly have strong views about the case it discusses and, if you read seriously, those views, whatever they are, will confront exceedingly uncomfortable counterarguments. You may then find the preceding chapters of some help in making your responses more rigorous, more aware of the strength of opposing positions, and less didactic. (As a bit of a pontificator myself I can confirm that critical or

vii

pontificate: to speak or express opinions in a pompous or dogmatic manner philosophical medical ethics is often unpleasant medicine—but it does ameliorate, if not entirely cure, the disorder.) To the sceptics who doubt the relevance of critical ethics to medical practice I recommend starting with the first chapter and then skipping to the chapter on "Conscience, good character, integrity, and to hell with philosophical medical ethics?". The former demonstrates the extraordinary variety of moral issues evoked by just one famous legal case in which a doctor was tried and acquitted of murder and attempted murder of his patient. The latter shows why it is not good enough simply to take each issue as it comes and rely on one's conscience, integrity and all that. To the abstainers I recommend starting wherever looks even vaguely interesting—but if you are not *totally* averse to intellectual challenge please go on to the last chapter! *I* certainly still find it uncomfortable.

In the course of the book I have tried to provide, following the admirable example of Beauchamp and Childress,[1] not only critical analysis, but also some argument in defence of four prima facie moral principles which seem defensible from a variety of theoretical moral perspectives and which I believe can help us bring more order, consistency and understanding to our medico-moral judgments. These principles—respect for autonomy, beneficence, non-maleficence and justice—plus attention to the scope of each of them—may not give us THE ANSWER to a particular medico-moral problem. But they can and do give us a widely acceptable basis for trying to work out our answers more rigorously. If, when confronted with a medico-moral problem, we consider the possible relevance of each of these principles to the particular circumstances then it seems to me that we are at least unlikely to omit any relevant moral concerns.

Some of the chapters are "heavier" than others, but despite the kind remarks of some of my medical friends ("couldn't understand a word—far too intellectual for me") I *know* that each chapter is comprehensible to the intelligent reader—provided he or she actually reads it. I know this not only because all have been read for comprehensibility by Richard Smith and Jane Smith, my patient and excellent editors at the BMJ, but also because each has been sternly screened for clarity by Angela Gillon, who is neither a doctor nor a philosopher, nor particularly interested in medical ethics (greater love hath no man than a wife who cheerfully gives up her book or her keyboard to read yet another draft).

To philosophers who may read this book I apologise for its over simplicity. Such apologies and attendant qualifications were recurrently chopped out of the text by the BMJ staff, on the grounds that the articles were not written for philosophers. Quite so—nonetheless I hope that they will read it, for I am sure that critical medical ethics needs further philosophical assistance, and my inadequate efforts may prompt better ones. Of course in America such philosophical involvement in medical ethics is now widespread, but in Britain there are still only a few philosophers who have grappled seriously with medical ethics. Quite apart from its benefits for medical ethics, such involvement may well help moral philosophy itself, which is surely likely to be enhanced by cooperation with thoughtful practitioners of a profession constantly confronted by moral dilemmas—often of great importance—which daily require practical resolution (or "closure" as the Americans say).

Finally my thanks to the enormous number of people who have helped me over the several years it took to prepare these articles. I originally wrote this preface naming the very many people to whom my debt is significant—but the length of the preface threatened to overbalance the book. In summary then, many thanks to all who helped me. Special thanks to my wife Angela for her great help, support and forbearance—it was a long haul. To my medical colleagues, including those I have met in the context of academic medical ethics who have pushed my thinking, and those around me who have tried so hard to keep my feet firmly on the ground of clinical practice, thanks too. My debt to philosophers, theologians and lawyers, both here and in America, is extensive and wide ranging, but to Michael Lockwood special gratitude. Many thanks also to Onora O'Neill, John Harris, Dick Hare, Robin Downie, David Hamlyn, Alastair Campbell, Kenneth Boyd, Gordon Dunstan, Jack Mahoney, Ian Kennedy, Roger Higgs, Douglas Black, Archie Duncan, and to other colleagues associated with the Journal of Medical Ethics, the Institute of Medical Ethics and the King's College London Centre for Medical Law and Ethics, interdisciplinary sources of much intellectual stimulus. My gratitude is also due to the staff of the Royal Society of Medicine Library, including those in the photocopying department, who have laboured so lengthily on my behalf. I dedicate this book to all who have helped me produce it, including my father who first set me on the path of critical thinking, and who has kept me at it ever since.

Reference

1 Beauchamp TL, Childress JF. *Principles of biomedical ethics* (2nd ed). Oxford, New York: Oxford University Press, 1983.

CHAPTER 1

An introduction to philosophical medical ethics: the Arthur case

In November 1981 a respected paediatrician, the late Dr Leonard Arthur, was acquitted of the attempted murder of a newborn infant with Down's syndrome for whom he had prescribed dihydrocodeine and "nursing care only" after the baby had been rejected by his mother. The complexity and difficulty of the case make it a suitable backdrop for this book introducing philosophical medical ethics.

What it's not

Rather than starting with an account of what I mean by this term I would prefer to start by stating what philosophical medical ethics is not. It is not the enterprise of quoting or even of drawing up professional codes of conduct. It is not an account of the legal constraints on doctors' behaviour in medicomoral contexts. It is not a sociological/psychological/anthropological/historical effort to discover the attitudes, mores, or ethos of a particular community, medical or otherwise. Finally, it is not the expression of religious rules or sentiments.

This is in no way to denigrate any of these activities. In particular, it is not to denigrate what might be called traditional medical ethics—that is, the long and honourable tradition in which doctors have established and promulgated among themselves rules and codes of behaviour considered to be morally binding. As I hope to show, however, philosophical medical ethics is additional and complementary to these other activities and ultimately can be expected to reinforce traditional medical ethics.

What it is

So what *is* philosophical medical ethics? Professor David Raphael gives a useful thumbnail account of philosophy as being "the critical evaluation of assumptions and arguments" and of moral philosophy as being philosophical inquiry about norms, values, right and wrong, good and bad, and what ought and ought not to be done.[1] In similar vein, medical ethics (I use the terms ethics and moral philosophy interchangably) is the analytic activity in which the concepts, assumptions, beliefs, attitudes, emotions, reasons, and arguments underlying medicomoral decision making are examined critically.

Medicomoral decisions I take to be those that concern norms or values, good or bad, right or wrong, and what ought or ought not to be done in the context of medical practice. At one level the purpose of philosophical medical ethics is simply to make such decision making more thoughtful and intellectually rigorous. Its ultimate purpose, as I (admittedly contentiously) see it, is to construct and defend a comprehensive and coherent moral theory for medical practice based on universal principles applying to all and capable of justifying particular lines of conduct in individual cases. This holy grail has certainly not been reached and may well be essentially unattainable. Perhaps the best that may realistically be hoped for are several competing theories based on widely acceptable principles. Either way, the activity of philosophical medical ethics is fundamentally critical; it lies full square in the socratic tradition that considers "the unexamined life is no life for a human being."[2]

The Arthur case

The first and crucial task of philosophical medical ethics (which I shall often call simply medical ethics) is to differentiate the issues.

The Arthur case manifests a quite remarkable variety of medico-moral problems, and in the remainder of this first chapter I shall try to untangle these. In subsequent chapters I shall analyse many of these issues separately, as well as some of the (surprisingly few) substantive issues in medical ethics that the Arthur case does not raise. First then, a brief outline of the moral "prosecution" and "defence" of the sort of treatment that Dr Arthur provided for the baby John Pearson. Although all the arguments I describe below were used either in the trial itself or in discussion of the trial, what follows is not intended, as I have indicated, to be a legal analysis but an effort to clarify the medicomoral issues raised.

THE MORAL CASE FOR THE PROSECUTION

The moral case for the prosecution runs something like this:

(1) All innocent human beings have a fundamental right to life; (corollary 1a) it is wrong to kill innocent human beings; (corollary 1b) it is wrong to deny innocent human beings reasonably straight-forward protection against life threatening conditions. Further-more, (2) doctors in relation to their patients, and parents in relation to their children, have greater than normal duties to protect the human beings in their charge. (3) It would obviously be wrong to give a normal infant who needed medical care nursing care only; even if rejected by his or her parents; this is (4) only morally permissible in some cases where patients are already dying. Similarly, (5) it would be wrong for a normal but rejected infant to be given a poten-tially dangerous pain killing drug when its pain or distress could be alleviated by feeding, comforting, and, in the case of chest infection, probably by treatment with physiotherapy and appropriate anti-biotics. (Illustration: imagine giving dihydrocodeine and nursing care alone to a normal but rejected infant distressed by three month colic, simple hunger or a chest infection.)

(6) It would also clearly be wrong for an older handicapped and rejected child, even one with Down's syndrome, reversibly un-conscious after, say, a road accident to be given nursing care alone or to be treated with potentially dangerous pain killers alone. Further-more, (7) distinctions between acts and omissions, between killing and letting die, could clearly not possibly justify such life threaten-ing treatment of normal rejected infants or of older rejected and handicapped children. (8) The newborn child with Down's syn-

drome is no less an innocent human being than are the normal newborn infant and the older handicapped child.

(9) As it is wrong to treat the older handicapped child with nursing care only and dihydrocodeine it logically follows that it is wrong to treat the newborn infant with Down's syndrome in this way, even if parental rejection has regrettably occurred. Furthermore, (10) under the law like should be treated as like; (11) as such treatment of normal infants or of older handicapped infants would properly be punished under the law so (12) it ought to be punished when meted out to rejected newborn infants with Down's syndrome.

That in summary is the moral argument of the Life organisation, whose members instigated the prosecution of Dr Arthur, and it would probably be the position of the Roman Catholic church and other orthodox religions, as well as of many other opponents of what Dr Arthur did.

THE MORAL CASE FOR THE DEFENCE

As for the defence, a composite summary culled from the trial and comment about the case runs something like this: (13) In general, a doctor's duty is to do all he reasonably can to preserve the lives and (14) restore or preserve the health of his patients. (15) He also has a duty to relieve, prevent, or minimise their pain and suffering. (16) In rare cases infants are born with such severe physical and or mental handicaps that medical intervention to increase the baby's chances of survival is not clearly justified. (17) Such lives, if they are preserved, are likely to be handicapped to a considerable and sometimes very severe degree and their chances of ordinary human flourishing are low. (18) Moreover, they are likely to impose a great burden of care on their parents (or other guardians) or (19) on the community if their parents reject them or die; also (20) other members of the family may be adversely and severely affected by this burden.

On the other hand, (21) some parents find the responsibility of this additional burden enriching for themselves and the rest of the family, and (22) some handicapped infants grow up to have very worthwhile lives. (23) In such variable circumstances the parents are the proper people to decide whether life preserving medical care should be given to the severely handicapped infant after (24) being given information by the doctor about the possible outcomes and their likelihood so far as these can reasonably be assessed. (25) It is arrogant and potentially cruel for doctors or anyone else to impose a decision contrary to the parents' own wishes in such circumstances, provided (26) there is no reason to suspect that the parents are incompetent to decide or (27) are acting maliciously. (28) Whatever their decision, the parents should be supported in its implementation and their suffering minimised. (29) If the decision not to employ life preserving medical treatment is taken the infant's suffering should also be minimised, and (30) pain killers and sedatives can properly be used for this purpose (31) even if they also increase the chances that the infant will die, for instance, by depressing respiration or appetite.

(32) A doctor must not kill his patient but (33) he is not obliged in all circumstances to prevent his patient dying. In particular, (34) he may in good conscience let severely handicapped very young infants die when their parents do not wish for life saving medical intervention. (35) Such cases are usually very distressing for all concerned, but (36) least distress arises if the decision making is left to parents in consultation with experienced doctors, all acting in good faith and mutual trust. (37) The addition of legal procedures and (38) the presence of potential spies from pressure groups can only serve to increase the parents' already considerable anguish and possibly also to increase the likelihood of the doctor practising "defensive medicine" rather than doing what he believes to be best.

THE ISSUES RAISED

I suspect that these two accounts of the rights and wrongs of the Arthur case incorporate between them the views of the great majority of practising doctors. They also incorporate a wide variety of substantive issues in philosophical medical ethics. Thus the prosecution's premise that all innocent human beings have a right to life (1), by making a rights claim (What are rights? Why should we accept that there are rights? Are there different sorts of rights? What follows ?), immediately elicits the fact that there are two major types of ethical theory. One type is based on rights and duties (so called deontological theories of ethics, from the Greek word for duty; much religious moral theory is deontological) and the other on the effects or consequences of actions (consequentialist theories of

6 PHILOSOPHICAL MEDICAL ETHICS

ethics, of which utilitarianism in its various forms is the main example).

Premises 1 to 6 in the prosecution's case all depend in some measure on acceptance of a deontological theory of ethics, as do premises 13, 14, and 15 in the defence. On the other hand, premises 17 to 22 all depend on consequentialist assumptions in that the happiness, distress, or flourishing (quality of life) resulting from an action are assumed to determine its rightness or wrongness. Both types of theory have major attractions and flaws.

The premise that it is wrong to kill innocent human beings (1a) raises the interesting issue of innocence and the crucial issue of what do we mean by human being in the context of moral reasoning. Do we mean any human being, from conception to cardiorespiratory death? any sentient (conscious) human being? any human being showing brain activity? Is there a morally important distinction to be made between a living human being and a living human person that might help us here? Clearly 1a is relevant to some of the most fundamental and familiar problems of medical ethics including those of abortion, euthanasia, and brain death.

Premise 1b, and more specifically premise 7, raise the philosophical problem of acts and omissions. Many, perhaps most, doctors rely heavily on the moral importance of this distinction in the context of killing versus letting die and it underpins premises 16, 23, 29, 32, 33, and 34. The profound question, however, remains: can a moral decision ever properly turn solely on the question of whether a person's behaviour is to be classified as an act or as an omission? This issue will be discussed in the context of two other doctrines of Roman Catholic moral theology often employed in medical ethics, notably the doctrine of ordinary and extraordinary means (perhaps hinted at in premise 16) and the doctrine of double effect (30 and 31).

Premise 2 evokes the issue of the relationship between people's general moral obligations and those imposed by their roles. For example, can it ever be right for a person to do something as a doctor that he would consider to be morally wrong in his role as an ordinary person? (What about a Roman Catholic doctor who refuses to arrange to perform an abortion but refers the patient, as is now professionally expected, to a doctor who has no moral objections?)

The whole argument (1-9) illustrates a basic method of moral argument. This is, to find a case or cases that are undisputed and argue that the case in doubt is morally similar to these and therefore should be treated similarly. Premise 10 alludes to the enormous philosophical problem of justice and 11 to that of punishment.

The case for the defence of Dr Arthur raises additional medico-moral issues. Thus premises 13, 14, and 15 imply that the moral foundation of medicine consists of certain duties; but in what circumstances do these duties apply? Again, what do we mean by "life" in this context, and by "health"? What sorts of suffering is it a doctor's duty to minimise?—all sorts?—and what is the relative importance of these duties, and how are doctors to choose between them when they conflict? Premises 17 and 22 provoke the question: what part, if any, should assessments of quality of life play in medicomoral decision making? Premises 18 to 21 raise the issue of how much the effects of medical treatment on people other than the patient should be taken into account: what, for example, is the role of the family and what is the role of cost benefit analysis in medical ethics?

Premises 23, 24, and 25 are highly contentious claims: should patients or their families, or both, make difficult and often anguishing medicomoral decisions that concern them or is this properly the responsibility of the doctor? Here the issue of personal autonomy is crucial; do people have the right (perhaps even the duty) to make their own moral decisions regardless of how difficult or distressing these might be, or should a doctor's duty to reduce his patients' suffering extend to diminishing their autonomy by taking such decisions for them? Associated with this issue of autonomy is that of lying to, deceiving, or incompletely informing patients in order to save them suffering.

Premise 34 raises the issue of conscience and 36 that of good faith, but what are these and what are their proper roles in (medical) ethics? The important question of the relation between law and morals arises in connection with premise 37, and 38 concerns the issue of what the Americans call "whistle-blowing": when if at all should someone who believes that an action approved and taken by fellow workers is in fact a heinous crime (murder for instance) "blow the whistle?"

Conclusion

The Arthur case thus provides a substantial basis for an introduction to philosophical medical ethics, and I shall pick up many of the issues raised in subsequent chapters.

It is vital to remember that the purpose of this book is not to promulgate a particular moral theory. It is simply to encourage more rigorous analysis than is customary of the moral dilemmas that confront all practising doctors.

We each must choose our medicomoral framework but, as with all other aspects of medical practice, we have a responsibility to choose critically, eschewing prejudice and rejecting slipshod, lazy, or incoherent reasoning. In this context the study of philosophical medical ethics can, I believe, be of some help.

References

1 Raphael DD. *Moral philosophy*. Oxford: Oxford University Press, 1981:1,8.
2 Plato. Apology. In: Jowett B, translator. *The dialogues of Plato*. Vol 1. London: Sphere Books, 1970:80.

CHAPTER 2

Medical oaths, declarations and codes

A common response to the new fangled concept of philosophical medical ethics is that it is unnecessary. Medicine has had its own scheme of ethics for at least 2500 years, and, although the moral rules of the Hippocratic Oath[1] have undergone considerable development and modification, much of modern medical practice is at least officially ethically inspired by its modern successors, the World Medical Association's declarations, including those of Geneva, London (the international code of medical ethics), Helsinki, Lisbon, Sydney, Oslo, Tokyo, Hawaii, and Venice.[1]

Declarations of the World Medical Association

The Declaration of Geneva (1948, revised 1968 and 1983) is a sort of updated version of the Hippocratic Oath. It requires the doctor to consecrate his life to the service of humanity; to make "the health of my patient" his first consideration; to respect his patient's secrets (even after the patient's death); to prevent "considerations of religion, nationality, race, party politics, or social standing [intervening] between my duty and my patient"; to "maintain utmost respect for human life from its beginning" (until 1983 the wording of this clause required "utmost respect for human life from the time of conception"); and not to use his medical knowledge "contrary to the laws of humanity."[1]

The World Medical Association's international code of medical ethics, adopted in London in 1949 and revised in 1968 and 1983, requires, among other things, adherence to the Declaration of Geneva, the highest professional standards, clinical decisions uninfluenced by the profit motive, honesty with patients and colleagues, and exposure of incompetent and immoral colleagues. It states that "a physician shall owe his patients complete loyalty and all the resources of his science"; and it says that "a physician shall preserve absolute confidentiality on all he knows about his patient even after the patient has died."[1]

The Declaration of Helsinki (1964, revised 1975 and 1983) governs biomedical research in human subjects, and among its many principles is the stipulation that "the interests of the subject must always prevail over the interests of science and society."[1] It also requires that in any research the doctor should "obtain the subject's freely given informed consent."

The Declaration of Lisbon (1981) concerns the rights of the patient. These are declared to include the rights to choose his or her physician freely; to be cared for by a doctor whose clinical and ethical judgments are free from outside interference; to accept or refuse treatment after receiving adequate information; to have his or her confidences respected; to die in dignity; and to receive or decline spiritual and moral comfort including the help of a minister of an appropriate religion.[1]

The Declaration of Sydney (1968, revised 1983), on death, states among other things that "clinical interest lies not in the state of preservation of isolated cells but in the fate of a person" and it stipulates the much more specific rule that when transplantation of a dead person's organs is envisaged determination of death should be by two doctors unconnected with the transplantation.[1]

The Declaration of Oslo (1970, revised 1983), on abortion, remains, even after its recent revision, which changed "human life from conception" to "human life from its beginning," the most equivocal of all these declarations for it requires doctors both to maintain the utmost respect for human life from its beginning and to accept that attitudes towards the life of the unborn child are diverse and "a matter of individual conviction and conscience which must be respected."[1] Subject to a host of qualifications the declaration has always sanctioned therapeutic abortion.

The Declaration of Tokyo (1975, revised 1983), on torture, is unequivocal in forbidding doctors to "countenance, condone, or participate in the practice of torture or other forms of cruel, inhuman, or degrading procedures."[1] It also forbids force feeding of mentally competent hunger strikers.

The Declaration of Hawaii (1977, revised 1983), on psychiatric ethics, requires inter alia: that patients be offered the best treatment available and be given a choice when there is more than one appropriate treatment; that compulsory treatment be given only if the patient lacks the capacity to express his wishes, or, owing to psychiatric illness, cannot see what is in his best interests or is a severe threat to others; that there must be an independent and neutral appeal body for those treated compulsorily; that "the psychiatrist must not participate in compulsory psychiatric treatment in the absence of psychiatric illness"; that information about patients must be confidential unless the patient consents to its release "or else vital common values or the patient's best interest make disclosure imperative"; that informed consent for the patient's participation in teaching must be obtained; and that "in clinical research as in therapy every subject must be offered the best available treatment . . . be subject to informed consent," and have the right to withdraw at any time.[2]

The Declaration of Venice (1983), the most recent declaration of the World Medical Association,[1] reiterates the duty of the doctor to heal and, when possible, relieve suffering and sanctions the withholding of treatment in terminal illness with the consent of the patient or, if the patient is unable to express his will, that of the patient's immediate family. It allows the doctor to "refrain from employing any extraordinary means which would prove of no benefit for the patient" and permits the maintenance of organs for transplantation after death has been certified, given certain conditions.

In addition to these declarations, the World Medical Association has issued other statements about medical ethics: on discrimination in medicine, reiterating its abhorrence of such discrimination on the basis of religion, nationality, race, colour, politics, or social standing[1]; on medical secrecy, affirming the individual's "fundamental right" to privacy[1]; and on the use of computers in medicine, again affirming the patient's right to privacy but stating that the transfer of information rendered anonymous for the purpose of research is not a breach of confidentiality.[1] Other statements concern medical regulations in time of armed conflict, family planning, 12 principles of provision of health care, pollution, the principles of health care for sports medicine, recommendations concerning boxing, physician participation in capital punishment, medical manpower, and medical care in rural areas.

The moral standing of the rules

Clearly the declarations of the World Medical Association contain a considerable body of moral rules that purport to govern medical practice. Why, however, should doctors take any notice of them? What is the moral standing of the declarations themselves? The question is given particular point as Britain has now left the World Medical Association having unsuccessfully tried to change its voting system to eliminate or reduce the ability of member states to buy voting power. Even if British doctors were morally bound by the Association's declarations when the British Medical Association belonged to the world body, now that the British Medical Association has left are they still thus bound? If so, why? If not, how can a change in medical ethics be justified on the basis of doctors ceasing to belong to a particular organisation?

One answer might be that the ethics of neither the World nor the British medical associations (as specified in the British Medical Association's handbook of medical ethics[1]) are the important ones. Instead, it is the General Medical Council's code of ethics, as specified in its little blue book,[3] that governs medical ethics in Britain because all doctors must by law submit to the General Medical Council's jurisdiction.

Is it then the law that provides a stable and coherent grounding for medical ethics? Surely not a stable grounding, for just as the World Medical Association changed its ethical principle from a requirement of "utmost respect for human life from the time of conception" to "utmost respect for human life from its beginning" so, considerably more dramatically, did British law change in 1967 from forbidding abortion except in the most dire circumstances threatening the mother to a law so permissive that many doctors understand it to permit abortion on request during the first trimester.

Sir Douglas Black, a past president of the Royal College of Physicians and a past president of the BMA, wrote that the change in the abortion law, occurring while he was a member of the

General Medical Council, whereby abortion "changed over night from being a crime to being something entirely legal, under appropriate safeguards" was influential in promoting his belief that "medical ethics are relative and not absolute."[4]

(More recently Mrs Gillick's success in the appeal court caused medical ethics as represented in the General Medical Council's guidelines on prescribing the pill to change. They changed again when the House of Lords reversed the appeal court's decision.)

Laws are not the basis of medical ethics

I shall return to Sir Douglas's question of relative and absolute ethics; certainly the ease with which laws can be changed, the wide range of conflicting laws that exists in different societies, and, above all, the powerful intuition that almost everyone has that it is possible for laws to be immoral all indicate that it is not law that grounds our ethics, medical or otherwise. Indeed, the *Declaration of Geneva* itself indicates that medical ethics is neither self sufficient nor entirely reliant on national laws when its pledges the doctor not to use his medical knowledge "contrary to the laws of humanity, even under threat."

The underlying assumption is that medical ethics is bound and justified by some more fundamental moral principles. What, however, are these "laws of humanity?" In the next two chapters I shall consider two types of moral theory—deontological and consequentialist—that attempt to answer this fundamental question.

The texts of all statements by the World Medical Association are available from the World Medical Association, 28 Avenue des Alpes, 01210 Ferney-Voltaire, France.

References

1 British Medical Association. *The handbook of medical ethics.* London: BMA Publications, 1984:69-81.
2 Duncan AS, Dunstan GR, Welbourn RB, eds. *The dictionary of medical ethics.* 2nd ed. London: Darton Longman and Todd, 1981. (See Declarations.)
3 General Medical Council. *Professional conduct and discipline: fitness to practise.* London: GMC, 1983.
4 Black DB. Iconoclastic ethics. *J Med Ethics* 1984;**10**:179-82.

CHAPTER 3

Deontological foundations for medical ethics?

In the last chapter I outlined the World Medical Association's principles of medical ethics and argued that all such codes, oaths, and declarations required some moral underpinning and that morally speaking they were not self sufficient. This was implicit in the Declaration of Geneva's appeal to "the laws of humanity." What, however, are these moral laws of humanity? Traditionally it has been the business of moral theology and its secular sister moral philosophy to try to answer this grand question, and, although moral philosophers have recently been rather more chary of attempting so ambitious a task, there remain strands even within contemporary moral philosophy that attempt to do so.

Among the diverse answers are two great categories of moral theory. One claims that answers to moral questions about which actions are right and which wrong ultimately depend solely on the nature of the consequences of those actions or proposed actions. Not surprisingly, this group of moral theories is called consequentialist, and its best known and most important members are those moral theories clustering under the name utilitarianism. I shall consider these in the next chapter. The second category of moral theories are the so called deontological theories (from the Greek word deon, duty, not from the Latin deus, god). At least some of the explanations of moral obligations offered by this group of theories

14

are not reducible to considerations of consequences.

Certainly most human societies rely in part at least on moral rules that make no reference to consequences, and it is widely accepted by psychologists that our moral reasoning is based at least in part on obedience to non-consequentialist moral rules instilled in childhood. The great religions expect obedience to moral rules (for example the Ten Commandments) that make no reference to consequences, and, as we have seen, some of the principles of medical ethics embodied in the declarations of the World Medical Association make no reference to consequences. None of this, however, shows either that moral explanation ought to be deontological or that these working moral rules cannot themselves be justified by reference to consequences.

How else then are deontological principles to be justified? Needless to say this is an enormous question with no simple answer. To offer any sort of outline account of one or two theories in a few paragraphs is bound to be inadequate and indeed to many philosophers offensively simplistic. Just as, however, kidney or liver function can be roughly explained in a few paragraphs for the benefit of philosophers who are interested, so too can the bare bones of philosophical theories be roughly outlined to non-philosophers; alas, here and throughout this series I offer no better and I hope that readers will bear this fairly limited objective in mind.

Two justifications

The great religions typically justify their deontological theories on one or both of two grounds. The first is that God has commanded the people he has created to obey his moral laws and it is their moral duty to obey their creator. The second is that the laws of nature include moral laws that bind everyone, including God. Even for believers there are important philosophical objections to the first position, for it commits them to accepting at least the logical possibility that if God were to command cruelty, injustice, or wanton destruction they would be obliged to accept that these were right and morally obligatory.

The second sort of religious justification, that morality stems from natural law, offers to religious and secular theorists alike a possible objective grounding for moral theories in "the laws of nature." In principle, at least, rational beings may be governed by their moral natures according to natural laws in the same way that the human tendency to walk on two legs and to understand mathematics is governed by natural laws. Attempts to make morality objective on the basis of such natural laws are, however, full of philosophical pitfalls including the ambiguity of the term natural law, and it should be added that there is little contemporary secular philosophical enthusiasm for such theories.

Kant's supreme moral law

Perhaps one of the most important non-religious deontological moral theories was constructed and defended by the Prussian philosopher Immanuel Kant. Although a devout Christian, he believed that an adequate theory of morality had to be justifiable quite independently of considerations about God's existence and also quite independently of considerations about mankind's inclinations, purposes, or happiness. Kant believed that the truth of his moral theory was a necessary consequence of the rational nature of human beings. He believed that he could prove that any rational being necessarily recognised himself to be bound by what Kant called the "supreme moral law."

This supreme moral law stemmed from the fact that rational agents (or persons) intrinsically possessed an absolute moral value (in contrast with inanimate objects and "beasts"), which rendered them members of what he called the kingdom of "ends in themselves." Not only did all rational agents recognise themselves as ends in themselves but, in so far as they were rational, they also recognised all other rational agents to be ends in themselves, who should be respected as such.[1][2]

THE THREE FORMULATIONS

The supreme moral law that encompassed this requirement could be expressed in three different ways: (1) The agent should "act only on that maxim through which you can at the same time will that it should become a universal law" (a maxim being any principle that in fact governs an individual's action or class of actions). (2) No person should be treated merely as a means but always also as an end. (3) The agent must always act as if he were a king creating a universal law for his kingdom of ends in themselves.

The first formula, sometimes known as the principle of universalisability, represents a fundamental theme within many different moral theories. The theme is perhaps most simply, though by no means precisely, expressed in the judaeo-christian golden rule, "Do as you would be done by"; or alternatively in its negative form, "Do not do as you would not be done by." This theme is also explicitly stated to be a component of utilitarianism by J S Mill.[3] But what seems to be crucially absent from at any rate most utilitarian theories is the Kantian claim that people have intrinsic moral worth that prevents their being used merely as means to an end (no matter how important or valuable that end may be).

CRITICISM

Kant's moral philosophy has been criticised for its excessive formalism, which some critics have misguidedly believed to have no implications for how people should actually behave. This, however, seems to be false. (One philosopher who is actively engaged in demonstrating the practical implications of Kant's moral philosophy is Dr O O'Neill.) Essentially, Kant's moral theory says act however you wish provided that your action conforms to the requirements of the moral law as represented above. The three principles (or as Kant argued, the single principle in its three guises; philosophers dispute their equivalence, sometimes vehemently[4]) undoubtedly provide important moral constraints in their demands for moral judgments to have universal application and for others to be treated as ends (what is sometimes called respect for persons).

Even if this is accepted, however, Kant's moral philosophy is rejected by some philosophers as offering far too austere, even arid, a version of morality in that it seems to have no central place for any moral obligation of beneficence, such as a positive duty to love others or at least to help them or to be in some way concerned with promoting their happiness. A further criticism is of Kant's absolutism, for Kant was unequivocal that the supreme moral law applied categorically, without exception.

Pluralist moral theories

Absolutism in the sense of relying on moral principles that apply without exception is a common feature of many deontological theories of ethics but not all. As we have seen, the various declarations of the World Medical Association contain absolute principles (for instance, that doctors must never take part in torture). Logical problems arise if a moral theory is both pluralist (containing more than one fundamental moral principle) and absolutist, if the principles can conflict. Suppose, for example, I accept the principles that I should never harm others and that I should never deceive others; if both principles are absolute and I am faced with a situation where somebody would be harmed if I did not deceive him I am logically incapable of acting rightly.

PRIMA FACIE AND ABSOLUTE DUTY

An important contribution to analysis of this problem was made by the English intuitionist moral philosopher W D Ross. He believed that the primary task of the moral philosopher was to list those moral obligations that on mature reflection we know ourselves to have. We find, he says, that there are quite a number of these and that they may indeed on occasion conflict. He thus distinguished between prima facie duties and actual or absolute duty.

Prima facie duties are those moral obligations that, if there are no conflicting moral obligations, we know should guide our actions. Ross described various moral principles that he believed any reflective person would intuitively accept: duties of fidelity (the obligations to keep promises and not to deceive); duties of beneficence (obligations to try to help others); the duty of non-maleficence (the obligations, more stringent than the obligation to help others, not to harm others); duties of justice (obligations to promote the distribution of happiness or pleasure in accord with the merits—probably meaning deserts—of the persons concerned); duties of reparation (obligation to compensate others for harms we have caused them); duties of gratitude (obligations to repay in some way those who have helped us); and a duty of self improvement.

According to Ross, it is self evident to any mature person on reflection that all these principles of conduct are prima facie moral obligations or moral rules of conduct that should undoubtedly prevail unless to obey them would result in a clash with some other rule of conduct. Although he did not claim that the list was exhaustive, he had no doubts that it was "correct as far as it goes," and that the "moral order expressed in these propositions is just as much part of the fundamental nature of the universe . . . as is the spatial or numerical structure expressed in the axioms of geometry or arithmetic."

What should be done when these prima facie principles conflict in any given circumstances? Ross did not believe that they could be immutably ranked or weighted so that we could know in advance which principles should take precedence over which. He also did not believe in any decisive overarching principle such as the Kantian supreme moral principle or the utilitarian greatest happiness principle by reference to which moral conflicts could be settled. Our moral life was far more complicated than the systematisers and simplifiers of ethics accepted, and when it came to specific cases of moral conflict we could only have opinions not knowledge about which principle took precedence.

Clearly it would be preferable to have some determinate procedure for resolving moral conflicts, but any decision procedure must, Ross believed, incorporate and reflect our basic moral intuitions. These were basic facts that any adequate moral theory had to encompass.[5]

CASUISTRY

In the absence of a determinate decision procedure the most common method for making decisions in cases where moral principles conflict is the much maligned method of casuistry, developed so exhaustively by both the Jewish and the Roman Catholic religions, also adopted by Kant, and also (in a way) by the British legal system. Essentially the method, whose objective is the application of accepted moral principles to specific circumstances in which these principles conflict, requires the careful separation of the moral principles relevant to a particular case, comparison with clearer or "paradigm" cases determined by each of the principles, and an attempt to settle the difficult case as coherently as possible with the existing pattern. Though the methods of casuistry have far more value than the common prejorative use of the term indicates, they are, none the less, radically limited so far as determining or questioning what those basic principles and their relative importance should be.

OTHERS

One further approach of pluralist deontological moral philosophers to the resolution of conflicting moral principles is to rank the principles in order of priority. For example, John Rawls, to whose theory I shall return when I discuss the principle of justice, argues for a "lexical ordering" of his two main principles, an order "which requires us to satisfy the first principle in the ordering before we can move on to the second . . . ."[6]

The questions whether a determinate method for resolving moral conflict is attainable in principle and has been attained are among the most hotly disputed in moral philosophy. In the next chapter I shall consider a cluster of theories that offer an affirmative answer to both these questions.

References

1' Kant I. Groundwork of the metaphysic of morals. In: Paton HJ, ed. *The moral law*. London: Hutchinson University Library, 1964.
2 Kant I. Critique of pure reason. In: Kemp Smith N, ed. *Immanuel Kant's critique of pure reason*, London: Macmillan, 1973.
3 Mill JS. Utilitarianism. In: Warnock M, ed. *Utilitarianism*. Glasgow: Fontana, 1974:268.
4 MacIntyre A. *After virtue: a study in moral theory*. London: Duckworth, 1981:42-5.
5 Ross WD. *The right and the good*. Oxford: Oxford University Press, 1930.
6 Rawls J. *A theory of justice*. Oxford: Oxford University Press, 1976:43.

Bibliography

Acton HB. *Kant's moral philosophy*. London: Macmillan, 1970.
O'Neill O. Consistency in action. In: Potter N, Timmons M, eds. *Morality and universalizability: essays on ethical universalizability*. Dordrecht, Holland: Reidel, (in press).
O'Neill O. Kant after virtue. *Inquiry* 1984;26:387-405.
O'Neill, O. The power of example. *Philosophy*, (in press).
Searle J. Prima facie obligations. In: Raz J, Ed. *Practical reasoning*. Oxford: Oxford University Press, 1978: 81-90.
Walsh WH. Kant, Immanuel. In: Edwards P, ed. *The encyclopedia of philosophy*. New York and London: Collier-Macmillan, 1967; vol 4: 305-24.

CHAPTER 4

Utilitarianism

There is something very attractive about the straightforward idea that morality is all about maximising happiness and minimising misery: that one's actions are right insofar as they tend to that end, wrong insofar as they tend to decrease happiness or increase misery and morally neutral insofar as they tend to do neither. This idea, encapsulated in the Benthamite slogan "the greatest happiness of the greatest number," is the basis of all utilitarian theories of ethics, which, though they have their origins at least as early as Epicurus, were developed by Bentham, Sidgwick, and Mill in the 18th and 19th centuries and have been elaborated and refined extensively by a variety of recent philosophers.

In my last chapter I discussed several sorts of ethical theory that reject the premise that ethics can be reduced to considerations of the consequences of actions, notably their effects on overall happiness and misery. Whether or not these considerations should be a necessary part of an adequate theory of ethics, the common theme of what I called deontological theories was that they were certainly not sufficient. Some of these theories, notably Kant's, were, like utilitarianism, monist theories in that they relied (or purported to rely) on a single moral principle. Others—pluralist theories—relied on more than one, potentially conflicting, fundamental moral principle. Moreover, some were absolutist theories in that at least one moral principle was held to apply categorically and without

21

exception while others were non-absolutist in that the principles were, as Ross put it, prima facie.

At first sight medical ethics, as reflected in the codes of such bodies as the World Medical Association, seem to fit well into an absolutist deontological ethical system for they contain some moral rules that apply without exception and that explicitly or implicitly reject considerations of overall happiness and suffering. For instance, the Declaration of Tokyo categorically rejects doctors taking part in torture. Some medical practitioners, on the other hand, see medical ethics as being basically utilitarian,[1] sometimes ruefully.[2]

In the rest of this chapter I shall try to outline the pros and cons of utilitarianism. Whether one ultimately accepts the theory (and I am inclined to reject even the most attractive version) it is important to understand (1) that utilitarianism has become a complex cluster of moral theories based on the principle of maximising welfare and that simplistic criticisms based on simplistic accounts of the theory are inappropriate and (2) that contemporary utilitarianism in several of its variants purports to encompass the ordinary prima facie "deontological" moral principles used in everyday moral and medicomoral decision making.

Advantages claimed for utilitarianism

Utilitarianism claims to overcome four major disadvantages of what I have called deontological moral theories. These are:

(1) The reliance on moral intuitions to identify moral principles notwithstanding the variability and unreliability of such intuitions. (For thousands of years intuition led people to accept slavery as being morally defensible.)

(2) The pluralism of many deontological theories, whose moral principles may conflict.

(3) The absolutism of more than one principle in some pluralist theories. If these principles apply without exception any conflict between them must be irreconcilable.

(4) Typically, the lack of a consistent and reliable decision procedure for choosing the right course of action in particular circumstances.

Utilitarianism purports to overcome these major defects in deontological theories in the following ways. So far as unreliable and variable intuition is concerned, Bentham believed that two moral intuitions were self evidently true and moreover accepted as true by everyone—namely, that suffering is an evil and happiness a good. He believed that from these two indisputable and undisputed facts the theory of utilitarianism could be derived. Moreover, as happiness and suffering can be understood to be poles of a continuum utilitarianism is in effect monist (based on a single moral intuition rather than two) and thus no pluralist potential for conflict arises.

Obviously there can be no problems of fundamental moral conflict in any monist theory, and in cases of apparent conflict (should one obey the law or steal to save the starving child ?) the quandary can and should be resolved by calculating the net effects of the alternatives on overall happiness and choosing the course that produces most happiness or least suffering (the so called hedonic calculus from the Greek word for pleasure).

The problem that arises when pluralist moral theories contain more than one absolute moral principle is also overcome for, although utilitarianism is strictly speaking both deontological (a duty based theory; one of Bentham's books is actually called *Deontology*) and absolutist, as it is monist there are no problems of moral conflict and, a fortiori, no problems of fundamental or irreconcilable moral conflict. Finally, utilitarianism claims to provide a consistent and reliable procedure for making decisions in one or other variant of the hedonic calculus.

If these claims could be sustained and criticisms countered utilitarianism would undoubtedly be an extremely attractive moral theory offering considerable advantages over pluralist deontological moral theories, but obviously there are important objections, and these can conveniently be considered in terms of the theory's coherence, its justification, and its results (see Bibliography).

Criticisms of the theory

COHERENCE

So far as coherence is concerned it is not clear what the theory is actually claiming. What for instance is the meaning of "the greatest happiness of the greatest number?" What is meant by happiness? How can happiness (and suffering) be measured? Is it total happiness, average happiness, or something else that is to be maximised? Finally, happiness of what?

What is happiness?—The Benthamite equation of happiness with (mere) pleasure was rejected early on by Mill, for whom the happiness to be maximised was eudaimonia or human flourishing. (As Mill put it, "Better to be a human being dissatisfied than a pig satisfied."[3]) Contemporary utilitarians, accepting people's variability, their powerful desire for autonomy, and their different perceptions of what it is to flourish, tend to aim to maximise satisfaction of individuals' autonomous preferences as being the best way of maximising overall happiness.[4]

Measuring happiness (and suffering) is clearly a major problem for utilitarianism, but modern utilitarians tend to agree with their spiritual accomplices, modern economists, in accepting that people can roughly measure at least their personal assessments of happiness and suffering[5] analogously to the way they can measure benefits and disbenefits in monetary terms (e.g. by buying goods or insurance policies and in their betting behaviour).

Maximising happiness—As for whether it is total happiness, average happiness, or something else that is to be maximised, a common response is to accept the widespread human concern with fairness as a fact about human nature and therefore aim at net average preference satisfaction as the appropriate goal. Its achievement can be expected as a matter of fact to maximise total happiness.[6]

Scope—The problems concerning to what or whom the moral theory applies are not unique to utilitarianism; deontological ethical theories may be just as troubled about how to incorporate non-human animals, very young human beings, and permanently unconscious human beings within their theoretical framework. Modern utilitarians tend to accept the (extraordinarily radical) Benthamite claim that anything that can suffer falls within the scope of morality[7] but they may accommodate the intuition that people are morally more important by differentiating according to the differing "interests" of people and lower animals.[8]

As for the somewhat abstruse debate about whether the scope of utilitarianism should include only existing sentient beings, existing and future sentient beings, or all possible sentient beings, suffice it here to assert that the problem is no greater for utilitarianism than it is for other types of ethical theory and that the most plausible option seems to me to be the second alternative. The first would exclude the moral interests of people who will exist but have not yet come into existence and the third would require moral consideration to be given to an infinite number of people and animals that will never exist. (This support of the second option in no way excludes from being morally relevant counterfactual consideration of possible people who might be affected by a contemplated action.)

JUSTIFICATION

The justification of utilitarianism remains a major problem. Bentham in effect merely asserted it, for even if it were universally agreed that happiness was a good and suffering an evil it would not follow that maximising happiness was morally obligatory or, even if it were, that it was the only, or the overriding, moral principle. Mill's notoriously inadequate quasi proof does not work either. (He argued that each person's happiness is a good to that person and the general happiness was therefore a good to the aggregate of all persons[9]). In more recent times Hare has offered arguments whereby he claims that a version of utilitarianism is derivable solely from an analysis of the meaning and logic of the moral words we use and in particular the word ought and its cognates.[10] Those who reject Hare's arguments may simply point out that the problem of ultimate justification is no more of a problem for utilitarianism (and no less) than it is for any other moral theory.

RESULTS

The third category of objections to utilitarianism comprises the counterintuitive results that it seems to entail. Thus if overall maximisation of welfare is the supreme moral objective the individual seems to be in permanent jeopardy before the overriding interests of society. The ordinary intuitive deontological moral principles that govern our relationships, such as respect for the integrity of each other's persons, for each other's autonomy, for promise keeping, honesty, and openness, for fairness and justice, and for the moral importance of special relationships, all seem disposable whenever overall maximisation of welfare requires us to ignore them.

Utilitarians have various defences to such criticisms, all turning on some variant of the claim that toleration of behaviour that ignores these principles is not conducive to maximisation of welfare. So called "act utilitarians," while judging each action or proposed action individually, in practice tend in specific cases to argue that adherence to conventional moral principles will in fact tend to maximise welfare. "Rule utilitarians" argue that even when the individual action may be expected to maximise welfare by contravening one of the conventional deontological moral principles the principle should still be followed because institutionalisation of such principles can be expected as a matter of empirical fact to maximise welfare.

J S Mill himself can be understood to have argued that the principle of respect for autonomy—insofar as such respect was compatible with respect for the autonomy of all—was a fundamental component of utilitarianism given that the exercise of autonomy was a prerequisite of human flourishing. Among the utilitarians who have done most to accommodate ordinary deontological moral principles within a utilitarian framework R M Hare is again notable.[10] (He also gives arguments whereby the distinction between act and rule utilitarianism in effect collapses and the insights of both are maintained.) In their helpful textbook on biomedical ethics Beauchamp and Childress (one a utilitarian, the other a deontologist) show how in practice both sides of this theoretical divide can agree on what might be termed working moral principles to be used in consideration of medicomoral issues.[11]

Conclusion

Of course, difficult philosophical problems remain. There are many utilitarian moral theories and not all are as sympathetic to the inclusion of deontological moral principles within their utilitarian structures as are Hare and Beauchamp and Childress. Most, however, have developed complicated ways of accommodating the standard deontological counterarguments to utilitarianism based on the counterintuitive results of a gross or simplistic version of utilitarian thinking, and in practice at least it seems to me that there need be no unbridgable incompatibility between non-absolutist pluralist deontological theories and utilitarianism.

(This article is based on my editorial in the *Journal of Medical Ethics* 1984;**10**:115-6. I thank the publishers for permission to use the material therein.)

References

1 Swales JD. Medical ethics: some reservations. *J Med Ethics* 1982;8:117-9.
2 Brooks SA. Dignity and cost effectiveness: a rejection of the utilitarian approach to death. *J Med Ethics* 1984;10:148-51.
3 Mill JS. On liberty. In: Warnock M, ed. *Utilitarianism*. Glasgow: William Collins, 1962:260.
4 Singer P. *Practical ethics*. Cambridge: Cambridge University Press, 1982:80.
5 Brandt RB. A defence of utilitarianism. *Hastings Center Report* 1983;13:40.
6 Smart JJC, Williams B. *Utilitarianism for and against*. Cambridge: Cambridge University Press, 1973:27-8.
7 Singer P. *Practical ethics*. Cambridge: Cambridge University Press, 1982: 49-50, 223.
8 Singer P. *Practical ethics*. Cambridge: Cambridge University Press, 1982:83-6.
9 Mill JS. Utilitarianism. In: Warnock M, ed. *Utilitarianism*. Glasgow: William Collins, 1962:289.
10 Hare RM. *Moral thinking: its levels, method and point*. Oxford: Clarendon Press, 1981.
11 Beauchamp TL, Childress JF. *Principles of biomedical ethics*. 2nd ed. Oxford: Oxford University Press, 1983.

Bibliography

Bennet J. Whatever the consequences. *Analysis* 1966;26:83-102.
Casey J. Actions and consequences. In: Casey J, ed. *Morality and moral reasoning*. London: Methuen, 1971:155-205.
Gray J. *Mill on liberty: a defence*. London: Routledge and Kegan Paul, 1983.
Miller HB. Williams WH, eds. *The limits of utilitarianism*. Minneapolis: University of Minnesota Press, 1982. (Bibliography)
Quinton A. *Utilitarian ethics*. London: Macmillan, 1973.

CHAPTER 5

Conscience, good character, integrity, and to hell with philosophical medical ethics?

One of the recurring themes at the time of the Arthur case was what a good man and doctor Dr Arthur was, a man of integrity. A recurring theme throughout medical discussion of medical ethics, typified by the British Medical Association's *Handbook of Medical Ethics*,[1] is the importance of recourse to conscience.

In addition to this positive attitude to the importance of good conscience, good character, and integrity, doctors often have a distinctly negative attitude to philosophical discussion, argument, and criticism concerning medical ethics. They agree with Dr Watt that too often it leads "to abstract and inconclusive intellectual argument—neither conducive to postprandial reflection nor necessarily relevant to the insistent demands on the busy practitioner throughout his day."[2] As for the possible role of medical ethics in medical education, many no doubt agree with Professor Swales that, "... ethical philosophy is qualitatively different from and irrelevant to clinical teaching."[3]

The argument against philosophical medical ethics

Often in conversation, though not often in print, clinicians can be heard to combine these two positions in the way summarised in the title. Slightly more fully the argument goes something like this:

There is something wrong with medical education if it has to go in for all this discussion and argument about medical ethics. (In my day) we learnt about medical ethics by learning to become good doctors, in all senses of good. We had had, I hope, good moral education, starting well before we came to medical school, at home, at church, and at school. Our consciences had been formed early on, and when we got to medical school the process continued. We learnt what was done and what was not done, mostly from the example of our teachers but also by firm reproof if we behaved badly or inappropriately, and perhaps we might even have been rewarded by a faint smile or a nod of approval when we did the right thing. At the heart of our medical education was an emphasis on character development, on personal integrity, on obeying our consciences—in short, on being a good chap. We never heard about utilitarianism and deontological theories of ethics or even about the virtues; we just learned what was appropriate in which circumstances.

I cannot pretend that this is a verbatim quotation from any particular doctor but I think it easily could have been and I should be surprised if it does not set many readers nodding vigorously and wondering if this will not have to be the last chapter in my book about philosophical medical ethics.

Why good conscience, integrity, and good character are not enough

My first and most important response is that I have never heard of any moral philosopher, and especially of any moral philosopher particularly interested in medical ethics, who is in any way opposed to the encouragement of good character, integrity, and a well developed conscience. What many philosophers are opposed to is any assumption that these features can be *sufficient* even for moral development let alone for medical or any other sorts of ethics. Personally I have no doubt that it is a necessary part of medical, and indeed premedical, education that students and doctors are educated to have a good conscience, a good character, and integrity, but as soon as attempts are made to explain what is meant by these qualities the need for some sort of additional critical philosophical analysis becomes apparent.

CONSCIENCE

Conscience, for example, turns out to be an ambiguous concept. On the one hand is a concept of an unthinking but morally controlling force within us telling us what we should and should not do. This is the concept corresponding to the Oxford English Dictionary's "internal conviction . . . the faculty or principle which pronounces upon the moral quality of one's actions or motives, approving the right and condemning the wrong,"[4] and corresponding to Freud's account of the "ego-ideal" or (later) "superego"—that is, the faculty of the mind in which the injunctions and prohibitions of "father . . . masters and others in authority . . . continues in the form of conscience to exercise the censorship of morals. The tension between the demands of conscience and the actual attainments of the ego is experienced as a sense of guilt."[5]

On the other hand is the concept of conscience corresponding to the Oxford English Dictionary's "inward knowledge . . . inmost thought . . . internal recognition of the moral quality of one's motives and actions."[4] This second concept also corresponds to many theological and philosophical analyses in which conscience is described as an essentially rational faculty; Father Gerard Hughes SJ, for example, wrote that conscience "is not the name of some privileged insight with which we were all endowed at birth and which functions quite happily ever afterwards. It is simply the name of our ability to reflect intelligently on moral matters,"[6] and in their textbook on medical ethics Beauchamp and Childress write, "In general, conscience is a mode of thought about one's acts and their rightness or wrongness, goodness or badness."[7]

It is thus immediately apparent that claims for the adequacy of a good conscience for medical ethics must make clear which of these two concepts of conscience is intended. If the non-thinking, non-rational faculty of conscience is intended the problem of conflict of conscience, whether intrapersonal or interpersonal, is left unamenable to reason. For example, if Dr A's conscience tells him to transfuse a Jehovah's Witness regardless of her own views and Dr B's conscience tells him not to transfuse such a patient, where stands medical ethics? Which position is right and why? Are both right? Why? Is no resolution or even attempt at resolution possible or desirable? Perhaps, it might be argued, a resolution could be attempted by appealing to good character and integrity, the two other members of the trio. They are considered below, but it seems difficult to deny the possibility, at least, that Drs A and B might both be of good character and integrity. (Were there not in fact doctors of good character, integrity, and good conscience on both sides of the Arthur dispute?)

The obvious way out of such an impasse is to choose the second concept of conscience, in which the exercise of reason is an essential element, but if that concept of conscience is chosen the original claim that moral philosophy can be dispensed with and medical ethics allowed to rest on conscience, good character, and integrity becomes vacuous, for "making reasoned judgments about moral questions" and "thought about one's acts and their rightness or wrongness" are the main constituents of the activity of moral philosophy.

INTEGRITY

With the concept of integrity there is again a preliminary problem of ambiguity: integrity can mean some morally specified and admirable condition such as "sinlessness . . . soundness of moral principle . . . uprightness, honesty, sincerity"; alternatively and quite differently it can mean completeness or wholeness. (Dictionary definitions such as these are rarely if ever of any substantive value in philosophical discussion but are often exceedingly valuable for showing that a word has more than one meaning.)

The usual sense of integrity relied on in moral philosophy leans on the second more literal concept of (moral) wholeness or of being one's own person. It requires identifying oneself with a particular moral stance and sticking to it in the face of temptation to abandon it; it also entails a sense of what one can and cannot live with and is thus a fundamental part of one's moral character and identity. This sense of integrity does not, however, seem to obviate the need for moral criticism, reflection, and argument any more than does reliance on one's (unreflective) conscience, for people notoriously vary in what they morally speaking can and cannot live with, and if impasse or war is to be avoided some sort of rational reflection is required. Furthermore, how is one properly to decide what sort of moral agent one ought to be, where one must say "enough, no further" without such reflection and criticism? Or should one, on the other hand, do merely what one was brought up and taught to do, without such reflection and criticism?

Surely even if the answer to that last question is yes it should only be given after such reflection and criticism. Iris Murdoch argues persuasively against the adequacy of such rational reflection and criticism, equating a Kantian rational agent with Milton's Lucifer[8]; MacIntyre argues powerfully for the importance of Aristotelian virtue theory[9]; but both of course recognise the need to provide philosophical justification and argument for their positions.

. The philosopher Bernard Williams wrote, "One who displays integrity acts from those dispositions and motives which are most deeply his, and has also the virtues that enable him to do that."[10] Here we have a concept of integrity that seems to use both the sense of wholeness and also some specific virtues akin to the first definition of integrity.

GOOD CHARACTER

The discussion thus shifts to the third member of the triad under consideration, good character or "virtuous" character. Can reliance on good or virtuous character (in association with good conscience and integrity) be sufficient for medical ethics and obviate the need for philosophical medical ethics? There seems to be two ways in which an affirmative answer might be plausible. The first is to claim that moral philosophy is primarily concerned with the virtues and therefore that study of different sorts of moral philosophy (for instance, deontological and utilitarian theories of ethics), is inappropriate. The second is to claim that doctors do not have to understand the philosophical underpinnings of their morality; they simply have to be of good or virtuous character.

Questions about the centrality or otherwise of the virtues are, however, philosophical questions. Thus even if it were agreed that moral philosophy is primarily about the virtues (a resurgent theme in contemporary philosophy) it would be absurd to suggest that this made it possible for medical ethics to do without moral philosophy; unless of course the claim is that, while *someone* may properly be concerned with critical study of the virtues, doctors need not be; they need only to be of good character.

Once again the problems of such a claim are unpacked along with the contents. What are the virtues of a good doctor? This is a question recurrently discussed by medical educators, and disagreement, as well as a wide variety of proposed answers, is characteristic of such discussions.[11-14] The idea that this question is not a proper concern of the medical profession is hardly likely to appeal to the sorts of doctors who claim that doctors need not be concerned with the critical study of the virtues, yet to answer it without such study—that is, without critical philosophical study of the moral assumptions and objectives of medical practice—is somewhat like specifying the syllabus for therapeutics while claiming that neither the medical students nor the doctors laying down the syllabus need know any pharmacology. Of course, such ignorance used of necessity to be the case in medical training, and we look back at those times with some regret. Shall we not equally look back with regret at our contemporary readiness voluntarily to eschew critical moral philosophy?

(Much of this chapter is based on my editorial in the *Journal of Medical Ethics* 1984; **10**: 115–6. I thank the publishers for permission to use the material contained therein.)

References

1 British Medical Association. *The handbook of medical ethics.* London: BMA Publications, 1984.
2 Watt J. Conscience and responsibility. *Br Med J* 1980;**281**:1687-8.
3 Swales JD. Medical ethics: some reservations. *J Med Ethics* 1982;**8**:117.
4 Little W, Fowler HW, Coulson J, Onions CT, ed. *Oxford English Dictionary.* Oxford: Oxford University Press, 1933.
5 Freud S. The ego and the id and other works, 1923-1925. In: Strachey J, Freud A, Strachey A, Tyson A, eds. *The standard edition of the works of Sigmund Freud.* Vol XIX (1923-5). London: Hogarth Press and Institute of Psychoanalysis, 1961:49.
6 Hughes G. *Moral decisions.* London: Darton Longman and Todd, 1980:26.
7 Beauchamp TL, Childress JF. *Principles of biomedical ethics.* 2nd ed. Oxford: Oxford University Press, 1983:265-8.
8 Murdoch I. *The sovereignty of good.* London: Routledge and Kegan Paul, 1970:80.
9 MacIntyre A. *After virtue—a study in moral theory.* London: Duckworth, 1981:216.
10 Williams B. *Moral luck,* Cambridge: Cambridge University Press, 1981:49. *See also* Williams B. Integrity. In: Smart JJC, Williams B. Utilitarianism for and against. Cambridge: Cambridge University Press, 1973: 108–118.
11 Crisp AH. Selection of medical students—is intelligence enough? A discussion paper. *J R Soc Med* 1984;**77**:35-9.
12 Linger M. Doing what "needs" to be done. *N Engl J Med* 1984;**310**:469-70.
13 Gelfland M. *Philosophy and ethics of medicine.* Edinburgh: Livingstone, 1968:54-60.
14 May WF. Professional ethics: setting, terrain, and teacher. In: Callahan D, Bok S, eds. *Ethics teaching in higher education.* Hastings on Hudson: Hastings Centre, 1980:230-3.

Bibliography

D'Arcy E. Conscience. *J Med Ethics* 1977;3:98-9.
Harris J. *Violence and responsibility.* London: Routledge and Kegan Paul, 1980.

CHAPTER 6

"It's all too subjective": scepticism about the possibility or use of philosophical medical ethics

In the last chapter I considered arguments that medicine did not need moral philosophy. Here I consider several common sceptical arguments suggesting that useful discussion about medical ethics is not even possible. Several of these arguments are variants of the claim in my title—that, unlike science, ethics of any ilk is subjective, a mere matter of opinion in which anyone's claims are as good as another's ("These are my ethics; what are yours?").

Perhaps one of the commonest variants is what I shall dub the argument from disagreement. According to this, although we all agree about objective facts—the sort of things that scientists are concerned with—we disagree radically across the whole spectrum of moral issues and such disagreements are irresoluble.

There are several sorts of counterargument to this position. The first shows that objective scientific claims are often themselves subject to radical disagreement, even within the scientific community. The second (which I shall not consider further as it seems obviously true) points out that disagreement in itself sheds no light on: (1) whether the disputed claim is true or false; (2) whether it is even

34

possible for the claim to be true or false; or (3) whether it is possible to know if the claim is true or false. The third sort of counter-argument is that in fact a wide measure of agreement exists about basic moral claims.

Disagreements in science and ethics

It is important, as the philosopher Renford Bambrough has pointed out,[1] to make sure that like is being compared with like when looking at the disagreements of ethics and science. Usually people offering the argument from disagreement compare a complex example in ethics with a simple example in science. Non-treatment of severely handicapped infants is, as I hope I have shown in my first chapter, a complex moral issue; thus it would not be legitimate to compare it with some straightforward scientific claim—say, the number of chromosomes characteristically present in human cells—and point to the widespread agreement about that. Instead, an appropriate comparison might be with scientific claims about the aetiology of cancers, the mechanisms of genetic expression, or perhaps the origin of the universe!

There are a host of radical disagreements throughout the sciences that are either explicitly admitted to result from ignorance[2][3] or are characterised by the sorts of disputed claims and counterclaims, supported by arguments and counterarguments, that are typical of radical moral disagreements. If such ignorance and radical disagreement do not undermine the possibility, use, or objectivity of science why should they do so for ethics?

It can, however, be argued that, although radical disagreement may exist about complex scientific claims, it does not exist about simple scientific claims but does about *all* moral claims. Well, consider the claims that material objects exist and that their properties are independent of our perception of them. If these cannot be classed as simple scientific claims what can? Yet, in addition to a long line of philosophers (of whom Berkeley is the best known[4]) who have contested them and given apparently cogent arguments for their beliefs, a contemporary theoretical physicist of repute has cast reasoned doubt on the existence of material objects, at least in anything like the form in which they appear to exist,[5] and has argued that many of our commonsense, simple beliefs about time and space are mistaken.

Other, less thoughtful, less reasoned forms of radical disagreement about widely accepted scientific claims also exist—for example, the opinions of the flat earthers about the shape of the earth. If the existence of disagreement in this case need not lead to scepticism or relativism about the shape of the earth why should disagreement about ethical issues lead to moral scepticism or relativism?

Moral agreement

To return to the third counterargument, is it *true* that radical disagreement exists about all ethical claims? Ignoring as irrelevant the fact that some people will always be found to disagree about any claim of any sort, ethical or otherwise, is there not in fact widespread agreement about the claim that it is wrong to inflict pain or harm or suffering on other people without good reason? That it is wrong to kill people without good reason? That it is wrong to deprive people of their liberty without good reason? That it is wrong to coerce people to do things against their will without good reason? The list could be extended.

I suspect that acceptance of such moral principles is widespread, not just in our society but in most societies (see various entries under anthropology in Reich's *Encyclopedia of Bioethics*[6] and Edel and Edel's *Anthropology and Ethics*[7]). Of course I have phrased the moral claims carefully, for it is perfectly clear that without the crucial rider "without good reason" the moral principles offered would not stand a chance of widespread let alone near universal acceptance. At any rate, the claim that radical disagreement exists about *all* moral claims seems highly implausible and, given the "without good reason" clause, the claim for widespread agreement about many moral principles seems at least sufficiently plausible to be worthy of appropriate empirical investigation however variable are the actual practices that acceptance of this (obviously by no means adequate or complete) set of moral principles may be claimed to require. It may be said, however, that it is precisely those variable practices that give the lie to my claim of widespread agreement about moral principles.

Bishop Butler somewhere wrote that it is in what people pretend that true morality may be discovered. When Hitler set out to wipe out the Jews, the Gypsies, and the mentally disordered he "justified" his actions on two moral grounds, the first being the crude utilitarian claim that the world would be better off without these groups, the second that the normal moral obligations preventing us from wiping each other out did not apply to these groups because they were subhuman, beyond the pale of our normal morality, and legitimately regarded as lower animals who might be destroyed for the benefit of those with full moral rights, the Herrenvolk. My point is that even Hitler and the Nazis, although they disagreed with most people about the moral acceptability of particular actions, accepted the need to give "good reason" for actions that would otherwise contravene moral principles to which they implicitly subscribed.

In general, I suspect that most people (with the probable exception of certain sorts of psychopath)—even the most evil people—would accept the moral principles I have outlined above. It is in their interpretation and application to practical problems that disagreement tends to arise. That is precisely, however, a part of what moral philosophy is about. Thus I conclude that the argument from moral disagreement fails to show that moral philosophy is either impossible or useless.

Radical moral sceptics

Sometimes one meets radical moral sceptics (especially in first year ethics classes) who purport to reject all moral principles. I do not believe that there is any satisfactory method of reasoning available to combat (philosophically skilful) radical moral scepticism (though as soon as the tyro radical sceptic indicates any substantive moral position himself—moral outrage, for example, at his teacher's proposal that all blacks or Jews or people from his part of the world should be excluded from medical schools—his bluff or confusion has been called, and moral discussion with him can begin). Furthermore, it is often remarkable that self professed radical moral sceptics who reject "commonsense" basic moral claims of the sort I have sketched above are perfectly happy to accept commonsense basic scientific claims. Before accepting their position we can reasonably request explanations of why if they accept the common-sense claims of science they reject the commonsense claims of morality; and, conversely, why if they reject the commonsense claims of morality they accept those of science.

Doctors' scepticism

Medicine being essentially a moral enterprise that aims to do good for others, doctors are almost never radical moral sceptics. Doctors' scepticism about ethics tends to centre on the beliefs discussed above, that ethics is a personal or subjective matter, that one doctor's ethics is as good as another's, and that there is no rational way to resolve moral disagreements arising in medical practice except perhaps by agreeing to differ.

This belief is too pessimistic. Although I am not one of those who believes that moral disagreement can in principle be completely eliminated, once moral dialogue has become possible as the result of some element of moral agreement (it may be no more than an agreement that it is a good thing to try to understand the opposed moral positions) considerable progress towards resolution can often be made simply by the use of careful analysis.

Such analysis may show that some moral disagreements are not disagreements at all; instead, usually because of the use of ambiguous terminology, the disputants are making claims that they mistakenly think are in conflict. (Two doctors may strongly disagree about the moral acceptability of "passive euthanasia" but on analysis realise that they both "let patients die" and conversely both "strive officiously to keep alive" in similar sorts of cases and for the same sorts of reasons.)

Sometimes the putative moral disagreement turns out to be disagreement about the non-moral facts of the case; for example, although some doctors disagree in principle with letting handicapped infants die, others who do not may in a particular case be outraged because they disagree with the assessment of the degree of handicap. They express their outrage, however, as if there were no moral meeting point between them and doctors who let handicapped infants die.

I suspect that in fact almost all doctors let or would let some handicapped infants die—consider anencephalics and other "monsters." The apparently clear cut and radical differences in principle between opponents over this issue usually turn out to be differences about what degree of handicap justifies such behaviour and why, and whether in a particular case the infant concerned has the relevant degree of handicap. Once the disputants realise this the impasse can often be unblocked and fruitful moral discussion pursued.

Analysis of the logical validity of the actual arguments used in cases of moral disagreement is also potentially fruitful. In their scientific discussions doctors rigorously eschew logically slipshod reasoning; yet it is remarkable how often logically fallacious reasoning underpins a medicomoral stance. But one example: one often hears the argument that as nature aborts a large proportion of chromosomally defective fetuses abortion of defective fetuses is morally acceptable. Of course the conclusion simply does not follow logically from the premise, and as soon as proponents of this argument are asked to supply additional premises to make the argument logically valid (for example, that everything that occurs in nature is morally acceptable) its weakness becomes apparent to its perpetrators.

A further potentially fruitful method of attempting to resolve moral disagreements is to try to confirm or refute a particular moral claim by considering its implications for other situations in which it should apply if the person making the claim is to be consistent. If, for example, it is morally acceptable to let newborn infants with Down's syndrome who are rejected by their parents die it should (unless other moral premises are to be added) be morally acceptable to let older children and also adults with Down's syndrome die if they are rejected by their parents.

Once again such analysis leads the perpetrator of the argument to seek additional premises to make his argument consistent with his other moral beliefs; if he cannot do so, if the necessary additional premise or premises would irresolubly conflict with those other moral beliefs, he may amend the second or reject the first. He cannot, however, if he accepts the need for moral consistency, maintain his previous position.

Conclusion

In conclusion, common arguments purporting to show that moral claims are essentially different from scientific claims in that scientific claims are objective and confirmable or refutable while moral claims are subjective, unconfirmable, and irrefutable do not stand up to criticism, and the same goes for several other claims purporting to show that moral differences are incapable of resolution. Scientific and moral reasoning are not as different as they are so often assumed to be.

This chapter relies heavily on Renford Bambrough's excellent book.

References

1 Bambrough R. *Moral scepticism and moral knowledge*. London: Routledge Kegan Paul, 1979.

2 Duncan R, Weston-Smith M, eds. *The encyclopaedia of ignorance*. Oxford: Pergamon Press, 1977.

3 Thomas E. *From quarks to quasars—an outline of modern physics*. London: Athlone Press, 1977:250-80.

4 Berkeley G. Three dialogues between Hylas and Philonous. In: Warnock GJ, ed. *The principles of human knowledge and three dialogues between Hylas and Philonous*. London: Fontana, 1962.

5 Davies P. *Other worlds—space, superspace, and the quantum universe*. London: Abacus, 1982:107-27.

6 Reich WT, ed. *The encyclopedia of bioethics*. London: Collier Macmillan, 1978.

7 Edel M, Edel A. *Anthropology and ethics*. Cleveland: Case Western Reserve University Press, 1968.

CHAPTER 7

To what do we have moral obligations and why? (I)

The moral prosecution of Dr Arthur began by claiming that innocent human beings have a fundamental right to life and that this entailed that it was both wrong to kill them and wrong to deny them reasonably straightforward protection against life threatening conditions (premises 1, 1a, and 1b in my first chapter). I shall look at rights subsequently. Here I wish to look at another profound moral question raised by these claims: to what do we have moral obligations and why? For example, and in John Harris's memorable phraseology,[1] by what criteria might we decide, on meeting a creature from outer space, to have him for dinner in one sense rather than the other?

If it is wrong to shoot peasants but OK to shoot pheasants this might be a matter that has nothing to do with the nature of pheasants and peasants; it might be an arbitrary (that is, discretionary) matter arising from some decision taken by people to allow pheasant shooting and forbid peasant shooting. Some moral obligations certainly do arise in this way. If I arbitrarily and knowingly promise to give Oxfam or the National Front £50 I am then morally obliged to honour my promise and this—assuming certain obvious stage setting—has nothing to do with the nature of Oxfam or the National Front but arises from what I have arbitrarily decided and under-taken to do. On the other hand, some of our moral obligations are, it seems fairly clear, not arbitrary and stem directly from the nature of the entities to which we owe those obligations.

41

Which entities are owed a moral obligation?

It is widely agreed (though it was not always so) that our moral obligation not to shoot peasants is precisely not the sort of moral obligation that we are free to accept or reject but that it resides in the nature of peasants, in particular in their human nature. Conversely, there is wide disagreement about our obligation to pheasants. Supporters of "animal rights" claim that the nature of pheasants is such that it does impose a moral obligation on us not to shoot them (or at least not to shoot them for fun: the claims vary), while those who accept the moral legitimacy of shooting pheasants argue that the nature of pheasants, unlike the nature of peasants, is such that shooting them (and again the permitted circumstances are disputed) is morally permissible.

The claim of the moral prosecution of Dr Arthur was that all innocent human beings have a moral right not to be killed and that this includes a right to some straightforward help in the face of life threatening conditions. Infants with Down's syndrome are undeniably innocent human beings and therefore have this moral right. Similarly, most antiabortionists argue that human fetuses and indeed all human embryos from fertilisation onwards are innocent human beings and have this right. Some supporters of animal rights argue that all animals have this right, and some people, who really do believe in the "sanctity of life," believe that all living things have this right. Indeed, this is an implied premise in some strands of Buddhism[2] and was central to the philosophy of Albert Schweitzer.[3] In all cases it is something about the nature of the entities that is supposed to ground the moral obligation we are claimed to have towards them.

Four moral positions

In this and the next chapter I shall consider four moral positions offered as justifications for differentiating morally between different sorts of beings because of differences in their nature. That is, I shall consider ways of deciding the scope of certain moral obligations, and especially the obligation not to kill, on the basis of the characteristics possessed by potential candidates for our moral concern. Obviously there are many more moral positions than the four I have chosen but these seem particularly relevant in the context of medical ethics. I shall also indicate some awkward implications of each of these positions, for I have yet to encounter a moral stance on this issue that is free from awkward implications.

Of the four positions I shall consider, the first is the Benthamite claim that all sentient beings (beings that can experience pleasure and pain) are morally equivalent and that whether or not to kill them depends entirely on calculations of pleasure and pain of all potentially affected. The second is that membership of the species *Homo sapiens* confers a unique moral importance and that all (living and innocent) human beings have the moral right not to be killed and the moral right not to be denied reasonably straightforward help in life threatening conditions (for brevity I propose to call all this "the right to life," though such abbreviation presents problems that I shall consider in later chapters on rights and on acts and omissions).

The third position is that all "viable" innocent human beings have this right to life and is commonly held by doctors who accept abortion but who also believe in the right to life of fetuses late on in pregnancy. The fourth, while usually accepting that sentience confers some moral importance, holds that within the class of sentient beings there is a morally more important subclass that possesses the special attributes grounding the unique moral importance due to people, including their right to life.

Sentience

Jeremy Bentham, a founder of modern utilitarianism, argued that sentience was the fundamental moral criterion and that all others were ultimately reducible to it. He believed that animals were morally equivalent to humans and that the utilitarian calculus, the basis of all morality, applied to them as much as to humans: "The question is not whether they can reason but whether they can suffer." He reflected that "the day may come when the rest of the animal creation may acquire those rights which never could have been withholden from them but by the hand of tyranny."[4] (Like many modern utilitarians Bentham actually thought that the concept of rights was nonsense, as we shall see in a subsequent chapter; but this does not seem to stop many such critics from using the term, usually, to be fair, in actual or implied inverted commas).

As I indicated in my chapter on utilitarianism, this simple claim that all sentient beings are morally equivalent is highly counterintuitive. Although most people would grant some moral importance to the need to avoid suffering and to promote pleasure, few are prepared to accept this as of equal importance in animals and humans, and few are prepared to accept it as the only or overriding moral obligation. Most people would argue that people are simply more important morally speaking than (other) animals and that this is so for reasons that are independent of considerations of pain and pleasure. How, however, are such intuitions to be justified?

Membership of the human species

One standard response, typified by Roman Catholic theology, is to claim that all innocent, living human beings from the beginning to the end of their lives are morally equivalent in having equal natural rights including an equal right to life. It would be a mistake to see this as grounded merely in membership of the species *Homo sapiens*; rather the claim is that all human beings who possess the morally crucial gift of a soul are in this special moral category and that their lives as human beings start at the time of this "ensoulment" or "hominisation."

When precisely it occurs is still today, as it has been throughout the history of the Roman Catholic Church, a matter of disagreement and debate. Current orthodoxy, though explicitly uncertain about this according to Father John Mahoney (the Second Vatican Council "deliberately leaves aside at what moment in time the spiritual soul is infused" and the Roman Congregation for the Doctrine of Faith acknowledges disagreement about this point and "does not proceed to ajudicate"), none the less requires Roman Catholics to behave as though it occurred at fertilisation and thus proscribes all abortion however early, including any destruction of the fertilised ovum before implantation by contraceptive methods having this effect.[5]

Mahoney himself, a Jesuit philosopher and theologian and a past principal of London University's Jesuit Heythrop College, argues that hominisation or ensoulment at fertilisation is highly improbable —rather it is more coherently understood as a process that must occur at or after the time at which (a) the developing embryo is no longer able to divide into twins (b) coalescence of embryos is no longer possible, and (c) cell differentiation rather than mere cell division has started.[6]

Other contemporary Roman Catholic theorists, deploying classical Thomist arguments, argue that hominisation could not occur until even later, perhaps after the development of neural tissue.[7] On the other hand, Iglesias[8] and also Grisez and Boyle in their powerful modern defence of the Roman Catholic "pro-life" position argue inter alia that any such theory whereby moral personality "joins" the developing human after its beginning at conception must entail a version of mind body dualism against which there are powerful philosophical arguments.[9] Roman Catholic counterarguments, however, to this claim by Iglesias, Grisez, and Boyle can either deny the need for dualism, using the Aristotelian theory of hylomorphism adopted by Aquinas whereby the human soul is seen as the "form" of a sufficiently complex human body (a form which a less complex human body simply could not have), or they can argue the case for dualism—no longer philosophically popular but still an option, as Eccles and Popper demonstrate.[10]

Such disagreements are not new in Roman Catholicism, for long ago that church's greatest philosopher, Thomas Aquinas, proposed, on quasi-Aristotelian grounds, that ensoulment does not occur until 40 days for boys and 90 days for girls.[11] None the less, there is no doubt that so far as practical issues are concerned it is widely accepted within that faith that all living human beings from fertilisation onwards are to be treated as morally equal and as possessing the full human rights possessed by all people, including the right to life.

A widespread moral intuition

Such a view is not limited to Roman Catholicism; certain protestants also accept it.[12][13] Such positions are not, however, generally shared by all protestant strands of Christianity,[14][15] by Judaism,[16] or by Islam.[17] In general, it would be fair to say that the stance of no killing from conception runs counter to a widespread intuition that newly fertilised ovums and developing embryos and fetuses are not in the same moral category as people and that unlike people they may legitimately be killed for the sake of (sufficient) benefits to others. Moreover, when the position that all human life has a right to life from conception onwards is combined with the view that man properly has "dominion" over (including the right to kill) other animals the combination also runs counter to an increasingly strongly held view that such a straightforward moral division between members of our species and members of other animal species is not morally defensible. How, however, are such moral intuitions to be justified?

In the next chapter I shall consider arguments for and against prohuman "speciesism," the claim that "viability" is a justifiable criterion for differentiating between humans that can be killed and those that cannot, and claims that "personhood" is the morally relevant differentiating concept.

References

1   Harris J. *The value of life: an introduction to medical ethics*. London: Routledge and Kegan Paul, 1985.
2   Edwards E, ed. *The encyclopedia of philosophy*. London: Collier Macmillan, 1967:1,417.
3   Schweitzer A. *Philosophy of civilisation*. Part 2. *Civilisation and ethics*. Chapters 19-22. London: A and C Black, 1929.
4   Bentham J. Introduction to the principles of morals and legislation. In: Harrison W, ed. *Jeremy Bentham's fragment on government and introduction to the principles of morals and legislation*. Oxford: Blackwell, 1948.
5   Mahoney J. *Bioethics and belief*. London: Sheed and Ward, 1984:52-86.
6   Mahoney J. *Bioethics and belief*. London: Sheed and Ward, 1984:67,69,85.
7   Donceel FJ. Immediate animation and delayed hominisation. *Theological studies* 1970;31:76-105.
8   Iglesias T. In vitro fertilisation: the major issues. *J Med Ethics* 1984;10:32-7.
9   Grisez G, Boyle JM. *Life and death with liberty and justice*. Notre Dame, Indiana: University of Notre Dame Press, 1979:375-80.
10 Popper K, Eccles J. The self and its brain. New York: Springer International, 1977.
11 Mahoney J. *Bioethics and belief*. London: Sheed and Ward:1984:58-9,71.
12 Stirrat G. From your letters. *Journal of the Christian Medical Fellowship* 1984;30:23.
13 Vere DW. Working out salvation: is there a Christian Ethic? *Journal of the Christian Medical Fellowship* 1984;30:14.
14 Dunstan GR. The moral status of the human embryo: a tradition recalled. *J Med Ethics* 1984;10:38-44.
15 Church of England Board for Social Responsibility. *Abortion: an ethical discussion*. London: Church Information Office, 1965.
16 Jakobovits I. *Jewish medical ethics*. New York: Bloch Publishing Company, 1975:273-5.
17 Musallam BF. Population ethics: Islamic perspectives. In: Reich WT, ed. *Encyclopedia of bioethics*. Vol 3. London: Collier Macmillan, 1978:1267.

CHAPTER 8

To what do we have moral obligations and why? (II)

In the last chapter I looked at claims that all living human beings have special moral importance including a "right to life" just because they are living human beings. I contrasted these claims with the Benthamite claim that all creatures that can experience suffering and pleasure are morally equal and that all moral issues including that of the right to life depend entirely on calculations of overall pleasure and pain, irrespective of difference in species. I shall now consider arguments about the moral importance of: being human; "viability"; and being a "person."

"Speciesism"

Professor Peter Singer, a contemporary utilitarian, argues against both the simple Benthamite moral equating of humans and other sentient animals and what he dubs the prejudice of "speciesism" (a neologism attributed to Richard Ryder and intended to be a pejorative term analogous to racism and sexism—"specism" would have been better). Thus, so far as pain and suffering go, Singer argues that "pains of the same intensity and duration are equally bad whether felt by humans or animals."[1] To be prepared to inflict such pain on animals but not on humans, other circumstances being the same, is irredeemably speciesist. On the other hand, argues Singer, human beings tend to have many interests that most other sorts of animals do not and cannot have. It is possession of such differing interests that can ground different moral rights and moral evaluation of human beings who possess these interests. Thus human lives that have a capacity for self awareness, ability to plan for the future, ability to have relationships with others and 'close family and personal ties, importance to other affected human beings, and other attributes such as the capacity for abstract thought and complex communication may, claims Singer, be legitimately valued more than lives that do not have these qualities.

This, he argues (somewhat contentiously), in no way undermines the principle that in making any moral decision the interests of all sentient beings affected by that decision must be taken equally into account; it is just that those interests are often vastly different. Such differences, however, are not determined simply by membership of a species. For instance, so far as a right to life is concerned "mere membership of our own biological species cannot be a morally relevant criterion. . . . A chimpanzee, dog, or pig, for instance, will have a higher degree of self awareness and a greater capacity for meaningful relations with others than a severely retarded infant or someone in a state of advanced senility. So if we base the right to life on these characteristics we must grant these animals a right to life as good as, or better than, such retarded or senile humans."[2]

Dame Mary Warnock doubtless speaks for many when she summarily rejects arguments against speciesism as "absurd." Such speciesism, she claims, far from being arbitrary prejudice "is a supremely important moral principle. . . . To live in a universe in which we were genuinely species-indifferent would be impossible, or if not impossible, then in the highest degree undesirable."[3] She does not, however, give much argument for her position and, like many doctors, she none the less wishes to differentiate morally between those very young human beings whom, or which, doctors are prepared to kill or let die in various circumstances and those to whom they wish to attribute a right to life that would prevent them doing so. Her answer is not quite clear but seems to require distinctions based on whether the embryo or fetus is (1) "plainly human" (in this context she offers as two exemplifying criteria the ability "to experience pain [and] to perceive their environment"); and (2) "a full human being" (alas, she does not say what she means by this). Over and above distinctions based on the nature of the developing human embryo or fetus she also puts great emphasis on respecting other people's moral outrage at any proposed action.

The trouble with all this is that in so far as it is clear it does not hold together. As Dame Mary writes, "human is a biological term"; but as such it cannot (in the absence of some additional moral criterion) give us a basis for the "supremely important" moral principle she desires. In any case, if her pro-human principle is to be understood biologically it will claim that all human beings are of equal moral importance, and this she clearly rejects. Furthermore, her criteria of experiencing pain and perceiving the environment cannot in themselves make the embryo or fetus "plainly human," either biologically construed (for many non-human biological species have these attributes) or morally construed, for there is nothing morally speaking specifically human about feeling pain and perceiving the environment. She may even be implicitly accepting such criticisms when she adds that it should be "absolutely prohibited" to anaesthetise the sentient human embryo for the purpose of experimenting on it. If, however, capacity for sentience and perception are to be her moral cut off points in the developing human embryo (1) she is no longer relying on specifically human attributes as she claims and (2) she offers no moral justification for rejection of the same moral cut off points in relation to other animal species.

Technical differentia

Dame Mary's dividing lines (if such they be) are among an enormous variety of such lines that have been proposed to distinguish morally between embryos and fetuses at different stages of development,[4] including the simple and widely accepted distinction between being unborn and born. Few, however, who think critically about the problem can justify this simple distinction (essentially based on the position of the infant relative to the mother's vulva) as being of moral importance.

A common medical fallback position is to claim that it is viability of the fetus that makes the moral difference. Before a fetus is viable it is seen as a morally acceptable candidate for abortion; after viability abortion becomes morally indefensible. (A less extreme version of this position has found its way into American law[5] via the Supreme Court's ruling in Roe v Wade.)

There are numerous problems with this position, among them the ambiguity, perhaps even incoherence, of the concept of viability. If, however, viability is taken to denote the stage of fetal development at which it becomes possible to maintain the fetus alive after it has left the uterus the alleged moral criterion turns out to be a (merely) technological criterion and a constantly changing one as medical technology makes it ever more possible to preserve the lives of premature infants. In theory any human embryo at any stage is viable with appropriate technology. Given the evidence of man's existing technological wizardry there seems to be no reason why Aldous Huxley's prediction of such complete mechanical incubation of human embryos should not become possible in reality, in which case the criterion of viability would collapse into the orthodox Roman Catholic criterion of fertilisation.

Viability, like so many other technical differentia, offers no (direct) moral rationale to justify treating previable human fetuses differently from viable fetuses. In any case, even without technology, are not most fetuses viable in the ordinary sense provided they are left alone to develop in the uterus?[6]

Personhood

So far I have suggested that a simple reliance on sentience, or on membership of the human species, or on technical differentia such as viability are highly implausible candidates on which to ground the scope of our moral obligations, including our recognition of a right to life.

In my earlier chapter about deontological theories of ethics I wrote about the radically different theoretical approach to problems about the scope of morality offered by Kant, for whom it was rational willing agency that afforded the moral criterion for distinguishing entities that had and were owed moral obligations from entities that were not. Such rational willing agents he called persons. John Locke, that most illustrious physician philosopher, also differentiated the "forensic" category of persons, to which praise and blame and other forensic attitudes were appropriate from other entities. Like Kant, and unlike many contemporary philosophers, Locke distinguished between the moral or forensic strand in the concept of a person and what might be called the ontological strand (ontology being the study of what is or what exists). While Kant saw rational willing agency as the essential characteristic of persons, Locke saw the ability to think combined with self awareness over time as the essence of personhood. Thus for Locke a person was "a thinking intelligent being that has reason and reflection and can consider itself as itself, the same thinking being in different times and place; which it does only by that consciousness which is inseparable from thinking and as it seems to me essential to it."[7]

One of the consequences of adopting either the Lockean or the Kantian criteria for personhood is that not all living human beings are persons. Embryos, fetuses, very young infants, and humans with severely damaged or severely defective brains may be able neither to think nor to be self aware, and if the Kantian requirement of rational agency is to be met many older children and some adults will fail to fall into the net of personhood. Yet the idea that a single living human being starts its existence not being a person, develops into a person, and then at some stage may stop being a person while remaining a living human being seems to be intuitively plausible both as an account of what happens and also as a basis for at least some sorts of important moral distinction. Indeed, it may be some such assumptions that prompted the World Medical Association in its Declaration of Sydney (about death) to assert, "clinical interest lies not in the state of preservation of isolated cells but in the fate of a person."[8]

Quite apart, however, from producing conflicting moral intuitions of this sort, the idea that living human beings can be persons at some stages of their lives and not at others produces many other sorts of philosophical difficulty, especially problems clustering around the concept of identity. Attempts to overcome such difficulties are legion in philosophical works and include three broad categories.

The first resorts to dualism, whereby physical bodies are understood to be composed of substances ontologically distinct from spiritual substances, minds or souls, with personhood being understood necessarily to require some non-material substance. (Descartes offers the classic dualist position in his sixth meditation, and Popper and Eccles argue for dualism,[9] though it is generally speaking out of philosophical favour.)

The second uses some variant of the identity theory whereby persons are identified with their bodies or some part or parts of their bodies, notably their brains.[10]

The third approach is to deny that personhood is an intrinsic property of any human being and instead to postulate it as a "social construct"—that is, an attribute socially conferred on some but not all human beings by other human beings.[11]

Problems with all these approaches are shown in the vast amount of philosophical writing discussing personal identity,[12] often by means of imaginary problem cases. These range from Locke's own example of the prince and the cobbler who swap souls and Shoemaker's modern analogue in which Brown's brain is successfully transplanted into Robinson's head (who is the result?) to real cases of the so called "multipersonality syndrome" and brain bisection at the corpus callosum with one half of the brain implicitly answering the same question differently from the other half.

Some philosophers have argued that the moral and philosophical problems of personhood are resoluble on the basis of the Lockean intuition that persons are essentially self conscious. Professor Michael Tooley, for example, has argued that self awareness is at least a necessary feature for being a person in the morally important sense of having a right to life.[13] As fetuses are not self aware they do not have a right to life. He confronts the obvious intuitive objection to this stance head on: newborn infants are not self aware either and therefore they too by parity of reasoning do not have a right to life and thus infanticide may be morally permissible. Tooley argues that, far from being a disadvantage of his position, this is a positive advantage in that it corresponds to a further widespread moral intuition; "most people would prefer to raise children who do not suffer from gross deformities or from severe physical emotional or intellectual handicaps. If it could be shown that there is no moral objection to infanticide the happiness of society could be significantly and justifiably increased."[14] He has recently changed his mind,[15] but the change is based on philosophically rather technical distinctions, and even under his new formulation persons necessarily possess, either now or in the past, a sense of time, a concept of a continuing subject of mental states, and a capacity for episodes of thought.[16]

Professor Tristram Engelhardt, an American physician philosopher, also argues that self consciousness is a necessary (though not sufficient) condition of being a person,[17] as does Professor David Wiggins (but in a very different way and for very different reasons).[18]

Among the many problems faced by this sort of position are the widespread and deeply felt intuitions (*a*) that newborn infants are of the same moral importance as the rest of us and have the same right to life; and (*b*) the slippery slope intuition that once handicapped infants are deprived of a right to life other infants and other handicapped people are at risk, as, ultimately are all human beings. Indeed, there are undoubtedly grave problems associated with any of these theories about what properties ground a right to life, and the problems are manifested particularly clearly in consideration of the moral standing of very young human beings, of live but brain dead, and live but permanently unconscious, human beings, and of animals of varying attributes. Although such issues have received considerable philosophical attention fairly recently, the subject still represents a lacuna in ethics as a whole and medical ethics in particular.

References

1 Singer P. *Animal liberation*. Wellingborough: Thorsons, 1976:19.
2 Singer P. *Animal liberation*. Wellingborough: Thorsons, 1976:22.
3 Warnock M. In vitro fertilisation: the ethical issues. II. *The Philosophical Quarterly* 1983;33: 238-49.
4 Veatch RM. Case studies in medical ethics. London: Harvard University Press, 1977:170.
5 Finnis JM. Abortion: legal aspects. In: Reich WT, ed. *Encyclopedia of bioethics*. Vol 1. London: Collier Macmillan, 1978:30.
6 Engelhardt TH. Viability and the use of the fetus. In: Bondeson WB, Engelhardt HT, Spicker SF, Winship DH. *Abortion and the status of the fetus*. Dordrecht: Reidel, 1983:183-208. This gives a slightly more sympathetic approach to viability as a moral criterion.
7 Locke J. *Essay concerning human understanding*. Book 2: Chapter 27, section 9. London, 1690.
8 World Medical Association. Declaration of Sydney—a statement on death. In: Duncan AS, Dunstan GR, Welbourn RB, eds. *Dictionary of medical ethics*. London: Darton Longman and Todd, 1981:135-6.
9 Popper K, Eccles J. *The self and its brain*. New York: Springer International, 1977.
10 Borst CV, ed. *The mind brain identity theory*. London: Macmillan, 1970.
11 Shorter JM. Personal identity, personal relationships and criteria. *Proceedings of the Aristotelian Society* 1970/71;1:165-86.
12 Rorty AD, ed. *The identities of persons*. London: University of California Press, 1976.
13 Tooley M. Abortion and infanticide. *Philosophy and Public Affairs*. 1972;2:37-65, especially at 44.
14 Tooley M. Abortion and infanticide. *Philosophy and Public Affairs* 1972;2:39.
15 Tooley M. *Abortion and infanticide*. Oxford: Clarendon Press, 1983:142-6.
16 Tooley M. *Abortion and infanticide*. Oxford: Clarendon Press, 1983:419-20.
17 Engelhardt HT. Some persons are humans, some humans are persons, and the world is what we persons make of it. In: Spicker SF, Engelhardt HT, eds. *Philosophical medical ethics: its nature and significance*. Dordrecht: Reidel, 1977;183-98, especially 190-3.
18 Wiggins D. *Sameness and substance*. Oxford: Blackwell, 1980:148-89.

Bibliography

Downie RS, Telfer E. *Respect for persons*. London: George Allen and Unwin, 1969
Vesey GNA. *Body and mind, readings in philosophy*. London: George Allen and Unwin, 1970.

CHAPTER 9

Rights

"All innocent human beings have a right to life," claimed the moral prosecution of Dr Arthur. In the last two chapters I discussed some of the problems associated with the term "human being" in this context. Here I shall look at some problems associated with the term "rights."

Essentially, rights are justified claims that require action or restraint from others—that is, impose positive or negative duties on others. An enormous variety of rights are claimed, ranging from so called human rights, via rights to unemployment benefits and free prescriptions, to the right to sit at high table or use the executives' lavatory.

To begin to make sense of talk about rights it is essential to make some distinctions. From the extensive variety of such distinctions that appear in philosophical and legal works[1-7] I propose to focus on two that are particularly important in this context. The first is between legal and other institutional rights on the one hand and moral rights on the other. Within the class of moral rights I shall try to distinguish between universal rights that are possessed by everyone and rights possessed by some but not all people either as a result of prior actions such as promising or making a contract, or arising out of special relationships or particular social roles. In the context of these distinctions I shall consider briefly what is meant by "inalienable," "human," and "fundamental" rights. The second distinction I shall consider is that between rights that require others to act and rights that require others to refrain from acting.

Legal and institutional rights versus moral rights

There can be no doubt that legal and institutional rights exist; examples are the various legal rights in Britain to free (that is, taxation financed) medical care, education, and other welfare services. As indicated above, a host of non-legal institutional rights are granted by many social institutions to their members or to certain subsets of their members. The common characteristic of legal and institutional rights is that they can be created and abolished by decisions made by the appropriate people, such as parliaments, committees, or dictators. Many would agree with Bentham that these are the only sorts of rights and that it is nonsense to talk of moral rights or natural rights (which, briefly, are moral rights "naturally" possessed by everyone), while the concept of inalienable or imprescriptible rights (rights that cannot be taken away from people) is "nonsense on stilts".[8] What reason might there be to disagree with Bentham's scathing rejection of moral rights?

Perhaps the most important is a powerful and widespread moral intuition that people simply have certain basic moral rights, certain intrinsic entitlements, that they can pit against any tendency of others who are stronger either individually or collectively to wrong them—and who in particular may band together to make laws and other rules that wrong them. The very idea that despots or despotic governments might decide to enact laws permitting (for example) the killing or enslavement or total dispossession of some group of people generally evokes a widespread and powerful moral intuition that, whatever the law may say, people have a moral right or entitlement not to be killed, enslaved, or totally dispossessed.

Such moral rights are claimed in various national and international constitutions: those enshrined in the French and American constitutions depend appreciably on the work of that distinguished physician and philosopher, John Locke. A powerful if at first surreptitious proponent of the English revolution of 1688, Locke was one of the most influential promoters of the concept of natural human rights, a concept that had had little place in moral philosophy until the late Middle Ages (indeed, it appears that the classical Greek philosophers had no word for rights[9]).

Interpreting earlier theories of natural law, notably that of Aquinas as providing "a complete equipment of human rights and duties,"[10] Locke defended the rights to "life, liberty, and estate" as being god given moral rights of man that people had a right to defend, if necessary by force. (Locke is often attacked for a "capitalist" preoccupation—that is, with the right to property—even though he explicitly states that he uses the term property as a shorthand for life, liberty, and estate.[11])

If one accepts the validity of such moral intuitions one is committed to the existence of moral rights. A remarkable cross section of moral positions do incorporate these intuitions including those of the "pro-life" campaigner, who believes in the right to life of fetuses or severely defective neonates, or both; the person who is against apartheid, believing that South African apartheid laws violate the equal moral rights to liberty of blacks; the libertarian capitalist, who believes that taxation violates the right to keep "the fruits of one's own labour"; and the marxist, who believes that capitalism infringes the right not to be exploited by others.

Others, however, reject the concept of rights or else, like some utilitarians, see them as a convenient fiction, general acceptance of which will tend to maximise welfare and is therefore morally justified. Non-utilitarian opponents of rights tend to accept the correlative moral obligations that human rights entail but deny any need to talk of rights on the grounds that the duties are sufficient on their own. They may add that emphasis on rights tends to encourage people to pursue moral demands on their own behalf at the cost of neglecting their moral duties.

Universal moral rights

If one accepts that people have moral rights it is worth distinguishing between the different sorts. One category is universal moral rights, which are attributable to all people or to all humans (hence human rights and hence various problems of scope as outlined in the two previous articles). Nailing his flag firmly to what some would call the speciesist mast of human rights, the lawyer Professor H L A Hart argues that if there are any universal human rights they are secondary to one fundamental human right (fundamental in the sense of not depending on some other moral right), notably the "equal right of all men to be free."[12] (Some would doubtless add the charge of sexist language to that of speciesism.)

It is clear from the context that Hart means, by right of everyone to be free, free to exercise his or her autonomy so far as this is consistent with everyone else's freedom to exercise autonomy. I shall return to the issue of autonomy in the next chapter, but the important (and of course controversial) point is that if there are any rights they all stem from the fundamental moral right to be an autonomous agent, which itself generates a fundamental moral obligation for us to respect each others' autonomy and thus accept restrictions on our own: a very Kantian position.

Special moral rights

In contrast with universal moral rights there are also (if there are moral rights at all) special moral rights possessed by some but not others. Some such rights arise from prior actions. Thus if Smith promises Jones £10 Jones has a moral right to be paid £10 by Smith. Fortunately for Smith this is not a universal moral right—though it is, as a moral right, universalisable in that anybody who has been promised something has a moral right to be given that thing by the person who promised it, assuming no disqualifying circumstances. (The importance of universalisability in the context of moral philosophy is clearly argued for by Hare.[13]) Contracts between people also create special moral rights, which are essentially based on reciprocal promising.

A second class of special moral rights are those arising from special social relationships, for example the rights of children to be looked after by their parents (genetic or otherwise; hence my suggestion that this moral right emerges from a social relationship rather than a genetic one). Hart plausibly argues that the whole network of our sociopolitical relationships is a source of special rights of which institutional and legal rights are examples; and the philosopher Professor Richard Brandt argues that all rights, including "worldwide rights" are a function of social systems.[14]

Types of duties correlating with rights

Some rights impose obligations on others to do things; others simply require others not to do things (apparently those that require others not to do things are sometimes called vested liberties rather than rights[15]). Rights to be paid are obvious examples of the first, the right not to be enslaved of the second. That rights do not of themselves impose obligations on the right holder, though he may also have an obligation to himself corresponding to the right, is worth noting. (Mill, for example, argued that there was not only a right not to be enslaved but also a duty not to sell oneself into slavery.[16])

An important question is whether there are, and indeed whether there can be, any universal rights that require others to act and if so which they are. Thus, although it is clear that the claimed universal moral rights to life, liberty, and estate impose a moral obligation on everyone to refrain from certain sorts of action, many find the suggestion implausible that they impose moral obligations on everyone to act and are not convinced that they require anyone to act. X's right to life, for example, clearly imposes a moral obligation on everyone not to kill X (other moral considerations not intruding); equally clearly it cannot impose on everyone an obligation to act to keep X alive. Is there, however, a universal right to life such that everyone has a right that at least someone else is morally obliged to act to keep him or her alive? If so how are those thus obligated to be identified and what is the extent of their obligation?

I shall not even attempt to answer these difficult questions here (though I shall consider them obliquely in a later chapter about acts and omissions in the context of killing and letting die), but it seems clear that if there is a universal right to life that morally obliges others to act positively to keep everyone alive (1) it is more complex than, and additional to, the universal right to life construed as a universal right not to be (intentionally) killed by others and (2) it has radical implications for most people's behaviour: the regular cheque to Oxfam is hardly going to satisfy its moral demands.

Finally, it is worth recalling that rights—even fundamental universal moral rights—do not have to be thought of as absolute. As I indicated in the chapter on deontological theories of ethics, absolutism has the consequence, untenable to many, that when absolute moral principles conflict it is impossible to act rightly; it is more plausible to think of absolute moral principles, including moral obligations to respect the moral rights of others, as prima facie absolute—that is, absolute when they do not conflict with other prima facie absolute moral principles.[17]

Undoubtedly, talk of rights can be transmuted into talk of others' moral duties: duties, for example, not to harm, to respect autonomy, to seek justice, and to help others. Rights, however, represent only a subset of the applications of those moral principles. One important differentiating feature of this subset is that it concerns situations in

RIGHTS 59

which it is morally respectable to *demand* from others a certain sort of moral consideration. It is this that helps to make rights so contentious.

Moral obligations are often seen as matters for a person to decide for himself. When, however, moral decisions lead to transgression of other people's rights such delicate non-interference becomes inappropriate. As Professor Brandt points out, the language of moral rights morally justifies, and indeed positively encourages, those whose rights are transgressed to feel resentment, to protest, to take a firm stand. Uncomfortable as this may be to others, it "hardly needs pointing out that encouragement of the oppressed and maltreated to stand up in their own behalf is beneficial for society in the long run."[14] Alternatively, as Professor Dworkin puts it, "Individual rights are political trumps held by individuals." They are crucial in representing "the majority's promise to the minorities that their dignity and equality will be respected."[18]

References

1 Feinberg J. Rights—systematic analysis. In: Reich WT, ed. *Encyclopedia of bioethics*. London: Collier Macmillan, 1978:1507-10.
2 Macklin R. Rights in bioethics. In: Reich WT, ed. *Encyclopedia of bioethics*. London: Collier Macmillan, 1978:1511-16.
3 Dworkin R. *Taking rights seriously*. 3rd imp. London: Duckworth, 1981.
4 Melden AI. *Rights and persons*. Oxford: Blackwell, 1977.
5 Benn SI. *Rights*. In: Edwards P, ed. *The encyclopedia of philosophy*. Vol 7. London: Collier Macmillan, 1967:195-9.
6 Frey RG, ed. *Utility and rights*. Oxford: Blackwell, 1984.
7 Finnis J. *Natural law and natural rights*. Oxford: Clarendon Press, 1984.
8 Bentham J. Anarchical fallacies. Reprinted in: Melden AI, ed. *Human rights*. Belmont: Wadsworth, 1970:32.
9 Golding MP. The concept of rights: an historical sketch. In: Bandman EL, Bandman B, eds. *Bioethics and human rights*. Boston: Little Brown, 1978:46.
10 Sabine GH. *A history of political theory*. 3rd ed. London: Harrap, 1971:526.
11 Locke J. Of civil government, two treatises. In: Carpenter WS, ed. *Of civil government by John Locke*. Vol 2. London: Dent Everyman's Library, 1925:159,180.
12 Hart HLA. Are there any natural rights? Reprinted in: Melden AI, ed. *Human rights*. Belmont: Wadsworth, 1970:61-75.
13 Hare RM. *Freedom and reason*. Oxford: Oxford University Press, 1963:2.2-2.4.
14 Brandt RB. The concept of a moral right and its function. *Journal of Philosophy* 1983;**80**:29-45.
15 Lockwood M. Rights. *J Med Ethics* 1981;7:150-2.
16 Mill JS. *On liberty*. In: Warnock M, ed. *Utilitarianism*. Glasgow: Collins/Fontana, 1974:236.
17 Vlastos G. Justice and equality. In: Melden AI, ed. *Human rights*. Belmont: Wadsworth, 1970: 82-4.
18 Dworkin R. *Taking rights seriously*. 3rd imp. London: Duckworth, 1981:xi,205.

CHAPTER 10

Autonomy and the principle of respect for autonomy

One part of the moral defence of Dr Arthur was that doctors should not impose their views on parents; rather, their role was to provide good expert advice concerning the various available options and then to support the parents in their decision, whatever that was, provided that the parents were not incompetent to decide and not acting maliciously. The claim rests implicitly on the principle of respect for people's autonomy. In this chapter I shall outline what is meant by autonomy and the principle of respect for autonomy.

A definition

Autonomy (literally, self rule) is, in summary, the capacity to think, decide, and act on the basis of such thought and decision freely and independently and without, as it says in the British passport, let or hindrance. (The word is sometimes used to mean other things as well, for example, moral reflection,[1] but moral reflection seems to be only one aspect of autonomy of thought and I therefore think it best to differentiate these concepts.) In the sphere of action it is important to distinguish between, on the one hand, freedom, liberty, license, or simply doing what one wants to do and, on the other hand, acting autonomously, which may also be doing what one wants to do but on the basis of thought or reasoning. Animals are not said to have autonomy but they may be perfectly free (at liberty), in what might be called the thin sense of freedom or liberty, if they are not constrained, for example, by cages, drugs, or having their wings pulled off by little boys.

Autonomy is a subclass of freedom or liberty, but not all freedom or liberty is autonomy. The concept of autonomy incorporates the exercise of what Aristotle called man's specific attribute, rationality.

Three types of autonomy

Autonomy is sometimes subdivided into autonomy of action, autonomy of will, and autonomy of thought.

Autonomy of thought embraces the wide range of intellectual activities that are called "thinking for oneself," including making decisions, believing things, having aesthetic preferences, and making moral assessments.

Autonomy of will (or perhaps autonomy of intention) is the freedom to decide to do things on the basis of one's deliberations. Although the idea of "the will" went into a phase of philosophical disrepute, it currently seems to be undergoing some sort of rehabilitation.[2] For the ordinary man and his doctor there is not much doubt that there is a human capacity corresponding to the idea of willpower (to the idea, for example, that one can decide to do, or not to do, something despite a powerful contrary desire and then act accordingly). Equally, there is little doubt that some people have more of such autonomy of will than others, that it is variable in all of us, and that it may be diminished by among other things, disease and chemical agents.

Autonomy of action—The patient whose voluntary muscles are paralysed by curariforms but who is conscious because his anaesthetist has forgotten the nitrous oxide and who tries in vain to devise a way of stopping the surgeon cutting him is perhaps a paradigm of a person whose autonomy of thought and will are active but whose autonomy of action is temporarily completely absent.

It should be noted that specific actions may be autonomous even though they are not the immediate or direct results of a thought process. One may drive to work perfectly autonomously without thinking what one is doing. One has, however, done so on the basis of reasoning, and one's actions are at any stage responsive to reasoning—one may, for example, suddenly remember the iron and decide to turn back.[3] Autonomy of thought, of will (or intention), and of action require some basis in reasoning.

Autonomy as a virtue

The philosopher Professor John Benson, in a stimulating paper on autonomy,[4] described autonomy as a state of character manifesting reliance on one's own powers in acting, choosing, and forming opinions. Seeing it as a virtue, he suggested, in Aristotelian vein, that it is a mean between, on the one hand, the deficiency of heteronomy in which one is excessively influenced by others (for example, by being credulous, gullible, compliant, passive, submissive, overdependent, or servile) and, on the other hand, the excess of arrogant self sufficiency or even solipsism (various doctrines exhibiting a total concern with self).

I am disinclined to accept that autonomy is a virtue—a villain is surely not rendered in any way virtuous by his autonomy. Rather, autonomy is a prerequisite for all the virtues in that these must, it seems to me, be based on deliberated choice if they are to be virtues. (That I take it is why the concept of virtue has only marginal applications to non-human, non-rational animals.) Whether or not this contentious position is accepted we can surely agree with Benson, and with the philosopher Dr Onora O'Neil,[5] that autonomy is a characteristic possessed by people in varying degrees.

The principle of respect for autonomy

Autonomy must be distinguished from what is often known as the principle of autonomy and which for clarity would be better known as the principle of respect for autonomy. It is essentially the moral requirement to respect other people's autonomy. In practice everyone accepts this principle to some extent: we all believe our own autonomy ought to be respected (who would accept arbitrary imprisonment without even a feeling of moral outrage?) and we are all prepared to accept that we ought to respect the autonomy of at least some others in at least some circumstances. In the case, however, of autonomy of action the need for some restriction on respect for autonomy is obvious; otherwise we should be morally required to respect any deliberated course of action no matter how horrible the results might be for others. How, however, are such intuitions to be justified?

Two great philosophers, one a founding father of utilitarianism, the other an exemplar of deontological (duty based) ethical theorists, argued for the moral importance of respecting people's autonomy and elaborated restrictions within this principle that, although expressed very differently, have perhaps some similarities. John Stuart Mill argued that to maximise overall human welfare respect for the autonomy of others was required in so far as such respect did not harm others and in so far as the people thus respected possessed a fairly basic level of maturity ("a capability of being improved by free discussion").[6] Immanuel Kant argued that both autonomy and respect for the autonomy of all other autonomous agents were necessary features of rational agency itself and thus of any rational agent. Let me offer crude thumbnail sketches of their arguments.

KANT'S ARGUMENT

Kant's metaphysics divides what exists into two great realms: the intelligible or "noumenal" world (the world of reason) and the phenomenal world of sense perception. In both realms everything that exists works according to universal laws.[7] Rational beings can act autonomously according to their idea of laws; non-rational beings are acted on, and their behaviour is heteronymous—that is, causally necessitated or determined by outside causes. Human beings are an amalgam of the rational and the non-rational, and it is the will that links these two aspects enabling people to use their reason to produce effects on the non-rational world, including the non-rational aspects of themselves.

There are various objective universal laws recognised by reason (think of mathematics and logic), and among these are a single moral law (which, as we have seen in the chapter on deontological ethics, Kant believed could be presented in three different ways). Expressed as the famous categorical imperative, it requires us to "act only on that maxim through which you can at the same time will that it should become a universal law." His argument in summary is that, as any objective universal moral law must apply to all rational agents, no maxim (principle on which in fact we act) could be consistent with such a law unless the maxim could consistently be willed by the agent to apply to all rational agents.

It is not sufficient, however, merely to act according to such a maxim; it is also necessary to will or choose to do so, for otherwise one is not acting autonomously but being acted on, and it is a necessary feature of rational agency that the agent acts autonomously. It is by both rationally recognising the validity of the moral law and willing or choosing to accept it for ourselves that we can be subject to the universal moral law and yet at the same time also authors of it.

Furthermore, because rational agents necessarily have wills they are necessarily ends in themselves, unlike entities that do not have wills and are (at most) mere means to an end. This, argued Kant, is true not only objectively but also subjectively in that rational agents necessarily conceive of themselves as ends in themselves. From the fact that people are ends in themselves and the categorical imperative it follows, argued Kant, that one must always "act in such a way that you treat humanity, whether in your own person or in the person of any other, never simply as a means but always at the same time as an end." Thus for Kant respect for autonomy was both a logically necessary feature of being a rational agent and also required that respect for the autonomy of any individual rational agent could be exercised only within the context of respect for the autonomy of all other rational agents.

MILL'S ARGUMENT

Mill also argued for the moral obligation to respect people's autonomy (except when to do so would be harmful to others), supporting this claim, as does R M Hare today,[9][10] on the utilitarian grounds that such respect would maximise human welfare.[11] Mill has traditionally been pilloried for trying to square the circle in endorsing both an absolute principle of respect for liberty (by which he clearly means autonomy) and utilitarianism, but the philosopher John Gray puts up a good case for Mill's consistency here.[12]

In the first place, Mill's "absolutism" is only apparent, for he builds in the qualification that respect for an individual's autonomy governs absolutely provided that this does not harm others[13] or deprive others of beneficial acts "which he may rightfully be compelled to perform."[14] In the second place, Mill may be interpreted as arguing that the principle of utility (maximising overall welfare) entails this respect for autonomy, for the welfare to be maximised is "in the largest sense grounded on the permanent interests of man as a progressive being."[14] Given that human happiness (in the broad Aristotelian sense of eudaemonia or flourishing) is constituted to a large extent in the exercise of people's autonomy and that people's autonomous requirements are so very different, indeed unique, it follows that respect for their autonomy will be at any rate a major obligation if the utilitarian objective of maximising welfare is to be achieved.

Bearing in mind the qualifications indicated above it is possible to understand how Mill as a utilitarian was able (arguably hardly less strongly than Kant) to advocate the principle of respect for autonomy:

"The object of this Essay is to assert one very simple principle, as entitled to govern absolutely the dealings of society with the individual in the way of compulsion and control. . . . That principle is, that the sole end for which mankind are warranted, individually or collectively, in interfering with the liberty of action of any of their number, is self-protection. That the only purpose for which power can rightfully be exercised over any member of a civilised community, against his will, is to prevent harm to others. His own good, either physical or moral, is not a sufficient warrant."[13]

In my next article I shall look at some counterarguments to this position.

I thank Dr Michael Lockwood for drawing to my attention the argument of A MacIntyre in reference 3.

References

1 Miller B. Autonomy and the refusal of lifesaving treatment. *Hastings Center Report* 1981;**11**:22-8.
2 O'Shaughnessy B. *The will: a dual aspect theory*. Cambridge: Cambridge University Press, 1980.
3 MacIntyre A. Determinism. *Mind* 1957;**66**:28-41.
4 Benson J. Who is the autonomous man? *Philosophy* 1983;**58**:5-17.
5 O'Neill O. Paternalism and partial autonomy. *J Med Ethics* 1984;**10**:173-8.
6 Mill JS. On liberty. In: Warnock M, ed. *Utilitarianism*. Glasgow: Collins/Fontana, 1974:135.

7 Kant I. Groundwork of the metaphysics of morals. In: Paton HJ, ed. *The moral law*. London: Hutchinson University Library, 1964:80.

8 Walsh WH. Kant I. In: Edwards P, ed. *The encyclopedia of philosophy*. New York and London: Collier-Macmillan, 1972:305-24.

9 Hare RM. What is wrong with slavery? *Philosophy and Public Affairs* 1979;8:103-21.

10 Hare RM. *Moral thinking: its levels, method and point*. Oxford: Oxford University Press, 1981:155-6,167-8.

11 Mill JS. On liberty. In: Warnock M, ed. *Utilitarianism*. Glasgow: Collins/Fontana, 1974:138.

12 Gray J. *Mill on liberty: a defence*. London: Routledge and Kegan Paul, 1983.

13 Mill JS. On liberty. In: Warnock M, ed. *Utilitarianism*. Glasgow: Collins/Fontana, 1974:135.

14 Mill JS. On liberty. In: Warnock M, ed. *Utilitarianism*. Glasgow: Collins/Fontana, 1974:136-7.

CHAPTER 11

Paternalism and medical ethics

In the last chapter I outlined different arguments supporting the principle of respect for people's autonomy and the Kantian requirement always to treat people as ends in themselves rather than merely as means to an end. An obvious and widely expressed counterclaim is that, although respect for autonomy may be important, it is often more important to do the best for people and especially one's patients—or at least to minimise the harm they suffer. To do this it may be necessary to override their wishes and to treat them merely as means to an end—for example, means to their own recovery.

Sometimes one has as a doctor to be paternalistic to one's patients—that is, do things against their immediate wishes or without consulting them, indeed perhaps with a measure of deception, to do what is in their best interests (see bibliography). Just as parents may sometimes have to make important decisions in a child's best interests against the child's will or by deception or without telling the child, so doctors sometimes have to act on behalf of their patients. As Dr Ingelfinger put it, "If you agree that the physician's primary function is to make the patient feel better, a certain amount of authoritarianism, paternalism and domination are the essence of the physician's effectiveness."[1] I shall look more generally at the principles of beneficence and non-maleficence subsequently; here I shall consider some arguments offered in support of medical paternalism.

67

Arguments for medical paternalism

The first such argument is that medical ethics since Hippocratic times has required doctors to do the best for their patients. The Hippocratic oath requires that "I will follow that system or regimen which, according to my ability and judgment I consider for the benefit of my patients."[2] It says nothing about doing what patients say they want, not deceiving them, consulting them about their wishes, explaining likely consequences, good or bad, or describing alternative courses of action.

Put so baldly this way of expressing the duty to do the best for one's patients may not sound attractive. Put in terms of various real life circumstances, however, with patients terrified by their diseases, perhaps suffering great pain and other highly unpleasant symptoms such as breathlessness, intractable itching, disordered sensation, misery and depression, and, often, utter bewilderment, it becomes far more plausible to think, especially if one is that patient's doctor, relative, or friend, that the last thing one should do is add to the misery and worry by passing on the results of the biopsy, the risks of treatment, the unsatisfactory options, or whatever other nasty bits of information the doctor has up his sleeve. More plausible indeed, but how justifiable?

Even if one accepts the claim that the overriding moral requirement is to do one's best to improve one's patients' health, minimise their suffering, and prolong their lives, it is by no means clear that these ends are furthered by, for example, false confidence, paternalistic decision making, evasions, deceit, and downright lies. Of course, such behaviour (the hearty slap on the back, "Well of course we're not magicians old boy but we'll do our best for you, you can rest assured of that, and we've had some excellent results . . .") greatly reduces the anguish for the doctor: honest discussions with people who, for example, have a fatal disease concerning their condition and prospects are emotionally demanding, as is the necessary follow up; it is far less difficult to "look on the bright side." The assumption, however, that this generally makes such patients happier is highly suspect.

What is more, it is often only the patient who is deceived and treated thus, while a relative or relatives are told the truth; the deceit that this imposes on the family (and also on other medical and nursing staff) may itself provoke considerable distress,[3] not to mention the breaking of normal medical confidentiality and the effects of doing so. Then there is the suffering of the patient who suspects that something nasty is afoot but cannot discover what. Finally, there is the suffering of a fatally ill patient on discovering that he or she has been deceived by his or her doctor and family.[4] What a way to go.

Of course, some patients really do want their doctors to shield them from any unpleasant information and to take over decision making on all fronts concerning their illness. Doing what the patient wants, however, is not (by definition) paternalism. My point is that not all patients want doctors to behave like this, and for those who do not it is highly dubious to suppose that their suffering is reduced by it or their health improved or even their lives prolonged. Skill, time, and effort are required to find out what the patient really wants,[5,6] whereas in practice it is often merely assumed that the patient "doesn't want to know".

A second line of justification of paternalistic behaviour is that patients are not capable of making decisions about medical problems: they are too ignorant medically speaking, and such knowlege as they have is too partial in both senses of the word. Thus they are unlikely to understand the situation even if it is explained to them and so are likely to make worse decisions than the doctor would.

Even if one were to accept that "best decisions" are the primary moral determinant it is worth distinguishing the sorts of decisions that doctors might be expected to make better than their patients from those where little or no reason exists to expect this. In the technical area for which they have been specially and extensively trained there is little doubt that doctors are likely to make more technically or medically correct (and hence in that sense better) decisions than their medically ignorant patients. The doctor who advises his patient that to continue her pregnancy would, because of coexisting medical conditions, be from her point of view appreciably more dangerous than to have a termination and that therefore a termination would be better may be giving medically sound advice based on superior medical knowledge. If he insisted or even advised that a termination would be better in some moral sense he would be stepping outside his realm of competence: he is not better trained professionally to make moral assessments than is his patient, and even if he were many would object that it is not the doctor's role even to advise on his patient's moral decisions let alone make them.

Doctors as assessors of happiness

The counterargument just offered meets the paternalist on his own ground by agreeing that there are some areas, notably the technical, in which doctors may be expected to make better decisions than their patients. It points out that in other areas, including the moral sphere, there is little reason to expect them to do so. A further matter on which it is doubtful whether doctors are qualified or likely to make better decisions than their patients concerns what course of action is likely to produce most happiness or least unhappiness for everyone, all things considered (the utilitarian objective).

Some doctors believe, for example, that in perplexing cases such as those of severely handicapped newborn infants it is up to them to "shoulder the burden," assess what course of action will produce the greatest benefit all things considered, and then implement it. As one paediatrician wrote, "In the end it is usually the doctor who has to decide the issue: it is . . . cruel to ask the parents whether they want their child to live or die."

The philosopher Professor Allen Buchanan has pointed out that if a doctor undertakes to assess which of various available courses of action (including informing the parents of the options and asking them which they favour) is most likely to produce the greatest happiness all things considered he must consider an awful lot of factors.[x]

"... [T]he physician must first make intrapersonal comparisons of harm and benefit of each member of the family, if the information is divulged. Then he must somehow coalesce these various intrapersonal net harm judgments into an estimate of total net harm which divulging the information will do to the family as a whole. Then he must make similar intrapersonal and interpersonal net harm judgments about the results of not telling the truth. Finally he must compare these totals and determine which course of action will minimise harm to the family as a whole."[9]

Buchanan makes a similar analysis for the doctor who tries seriously to assess whether it would be best, all things considered, to tell a dying patient the truth about his predicament. After showing the complexity of any such analysis and its necessarily morally evaluative components Buchanan concludes:

"Furthermore, once the complexity of these judgments is appreciated and once their evaluative character is understood it is implausible to hold that the physician is in a better position to make them than the patient or his family. The failure to ask what sorts of harm/benefit judgments may properly be made by the physician in his capacity as a physician is a fundamental feature of medical paternalism."[10]

Of course, such assessments—moral and preference assessments—are difficult for anyone to make. The point is that there is no prima facie reason to suppose that doctors make them better than their patients. Even in the strongest case, that of technical medical assessments, the argument from patient ignorance is suspect for in practice many doctors can explain technical medical issues to their patients' satisfaction. Better postgraduate training in effective communication or delegation to colleagues who have these skills, or both, are alternatives to arguing that such effective communication cannot be achieved.

All the preceding counterarguments meet the defence of paternalism on its own ground by accepting its assumption that the overriding moral objective is to maximise the happiness of the patient alone, of the family, or of society as a whole. Kantians (for whom the principle of respect for autonomy is morally supreme) and pluralist deontologists (who believe that an adequate moral theory requires a variety of potentially conflicting moral principles including that of respect for autonomy) will argue that there are many circumstances in which a person's autonomy must be respected even if to do so will result in an obviously worse decision in terms of the patient's, the family's, or, even, a particular society's happiness. And as we have seen in the last chapter as well as in the chapter on utilitarianism, this conclusion is also supported by many utilitarians on the grounds that respect for people's autonomy is required if human welfare really is to be maximised.[11-15]

Sir Richard Bayliss has movingly described the case of a Christian Scientist whose decision to turn to orthodox medicine for treatment of her thyrotoxicosis came too late to save her life[16]. Few who do not accept Christian Scientism can believe she made a "better" decision in relation to her longevity and health when she rejected the advice of her original doctor in favour of her cult's. Those, however, for whom the principle of respect for autonomy is morally important would not deny her the respect of allowing her to refuse medical help in the first place even though this was highly likely to be fatal and thus cause her family and medical attendants great anguish and even though paternalistic intervention could have saved her life.

References

1 Ingelfinger FJ. Arrogance. *N Engl J Med* 1980;**303**:1507-11.
2 British Medical Association. *The handbook of medical ethics.* London: BMA, 1984:69-70.
3 Kubler-Ross E. *On death and dying.* London: Tavistock Publications, 1970:149-50.
4 Kubler-Ross E. *On death and dying.* London: Tavistock Publications, 1970:32.
5 Nicholls J. Patients too timid to ask questions of their GPs. *Medical News* 1982 July 1:23.
6 Hull FM, Hull FS. Time and the general practitioner: the patient's view. *J R Coll Gen Pract* 1984;**34**:71-5.
7 Shaw A, Shaw I. Dilemmas of "informed consent" in children. *N Engl J Med* 1973;**289**:885-90.
8 Buchanan A. Medical paternalism. *Philosophy and Public Affairs* 1978;7:370-90.
9 Buchanan A. Medical paternalism. *Philosophy and Public Affairs* 1978;7:380.
10 Buchanan A. Medical paternalism. *Philosophy and Public Affairs* 1978;7:383.
11 Mill JS. On liberty. In: Warnock M, ed. Utilitarianism. Glasgow: Collins/Fontana, 1974.
12 Hare RM. Ethical theory and utilitarianism. In: Lewis HD, ed. *Contemporary moral philosophy 4.* London: Allen and Unwin, 1976.
13 Hare RM. *Moral thinking—its levels, method and point.* Oxford: Clarendon Press, 1981.
14 Singer P. *Practical ethics.* Cambridge: Cambridge University Press, 1979:72-92, 140-6.
15 Haworth L. Autonomy and utility. *Ethics* 1984;**95**:5-19.
16 Bayliss R. A health hazard. *Br Med J* 1982;**285**:1824-5.

Bibliography

Accounts of paternalism

Gorovitz S, Jameton AL, Macklin R, *et al. Moral problems in medicine.* 1st ed. Englewood Cliffs: Prentice-Hall, 1976:182-241.
Culver CM, Gert D. *Philosophy in medicine—conceptual and ethical issues in medicine and psychiatry.* New York/Oxford: Oxford University Press, 1982:126-63.
Sartorius RE, ed. *Paternalism.* Minneapolis: University of Minnesota Press, 1983.

CHAPTER 12

Beneficence: doing good for others

Among the more pious remarks to be heard in discussion of medical ethics is, "The patient's interests always come first." It takes only a few moments of reflection to see that this is certainly not true in practice and undesirable as a moral imperative. There are many competing interests in a person's life, including his own and those of his loved ones, the interests of those to whom he has special obligations, and the interests of his community. In the context of such conflict of interest it is, generally at any rate, unthinking absolutism to state that any one person's or group's interests always come first. Indeed, the extent to which beneficence or doing good for others is morally obligatory is vigorously debated by moral theorists[1] (see bibliography), and some even argue that there is no such moral obligation, though they usually hasten to add that beneficence is undoubtedly a virtue and morally commendable.[2]

Whatever the case in general ethics, it is undoubtedly true that members of the medical profession undertake to place the interests of their patients before their own in many circumstances. This undertaking differentiates them from, for instance, merchants, who, while they may also on occasion put their clients' interests first, will do so (qua merchants) only to further their own longer term interests—for example, when it is good for business to put themselves out for their clients. Although an element of such self interest undoubtedly exists in the practice of medicine and although the grandiose claim that interests of patients always come first is false as a description and undesirable as a prescription, the medical profession none the less conceives itself, and is conceived by society, as having a duty of beneficence to the sick in general and to its patients in particular. One does not hear the Tannoy ringing out during a ball with the request, "Would any architect present please report to the manager's office"; and if one did no architect there would feel the slightest moral obligation to respond.

The source of this additional moral obligation of beneficence taken on by doctors is presumably a certain feeling of benevolence, good will, or sympathy towards the sick. No doubt there are some who go into medicine only for the money, power, and prestige, and perhaps these factors are part of the motivation for most, but there cannot be many who do not at least start off their medical careers with a large measure of sympathy for people afflicted by illness and a desire to commit their working lives to helping them. If, however, such benevolence is to result in real beneficence—that is, doing good rather than, for instance, merely feeling good, do-gooding, meddling, or even behaving unjustly—various constraints apply.

Constraints to beneficence

Three important constraints are: (1) The need to respect the autonomy of those whom one intends to help, especially to find out what it is they want in the way of help (the duty of beneficence needs to be tempered by the duty of respect for autonomy). (2) The need to ensure that the help one renders is not bought at too high a price (the duty of beneficence needs to be tempered by the duty of non-maleficence). (3) The need to consider the wants, needs, and rights of others (the duty of beneficence must be tempered by the duty of justice).

THE DUTY OF RESPECT FOR AUTONOMY

In previous chapters on autonomy and medical paternalism I have argued that in general autonomy, when it exists, ought to be respected in so far as such respect is compatible with respect for the autonomy of others. In a subsequent chapter I shall consider circumstances in which the presumption of beneficence supersedes the presumption of respect for autonomy. In most cases, however, of a doctor's dealings with patients (or clients—they are not always patients) not only is there an independent moral presumption that he must respect their autonomy but, even if he is interested only in doing them good, he must generally respect their autonomy in order to do so.

If one wants to do good for a patient or client one generally needs to find out what he or she actually wants one to do. Often this does not need much inquiry; a person who has broken his arm wants it set and the pain relieved. Doctors, however, are often too ready to assume that they can tell what the patient wants, or even what is best for the patient, without asking. In even the simplest of interactions patients in similar circumstances want different things from their doctors. One patient with a sore throat wants antibiotics, another wants a pain killer, a third wants information about what it is, whether it is likely to go to his chest, whether deterioration can be prevented, and if so how, and a fourth wants a sick note for his employer but refuses treatment, preferring to let nature take its course. The doctor who "knows" what the patient wants without asking him is quite likely to get it wrong.

Sometimes it is true that patients' wants and needs may be in conflict. The patient who wants antibiotics for his sore throat may be wanting something that will not benefit him—for example, if he or she has a viral infection, as is commonly the case. Conversely, he may want not to have what will benefit him (as when a patient with a persistent, confirmed pathogenic streptococcal infection refuses penicillin—"I can't abide antibiotics"—and risks heart and kidney damage). In each case the duty of beneficence requires at least discovery of what the patient does want and an explanation of why a different course of action would probably (for almost all such assessments are probabilistic) benefit him more. Such respect, even if an independent priority to respect for autonomy is rejected, is required by beneficence simply because the patient is more likely to do what the doctor considers to be medically optimal if the doctor explains why the patient's own preference is less likely to be beneficial. Conversely, the doctor is more likely to make a truly beneficial proposal if he knows and takes into account the patient's own preferences.

The doctor is not obliged by the (prima facie) duty of beneficence always to do what the patient after such discussion wants. Self respect for one's own moral autonomy is properly part of the moral assessment, and there are some actions that one may properly refuse to take because they go against one's own moral principles: one may believe, whether or not the person concerned agrees, that they would be too harmful; one may wish to respect the law or one's professional code of ethics; or one may consider them unjust even if they will benefit the patient. Prescription of an expensive drug preferred by the patient when there is good reason to believe that a cheaper one is likely to be just as effective is, at least when others are paying, ultimately unjust for it places unnecessary and therefore excessive burdens on those others (taxpayers, contributors to insurance schemes, or charitable benefactors). Similarly, the provision of as much time for discussion as the patient (and doctor) may like may be unjust in depriving other patients of adequate time in their turn. None of that, however, negates the prima facie requirement of the obligation of beneficence to find out what the patient wants and to try to meet those requirements.

THE DUTY TO DO NO HARM

A second moral obligation that must necessarily temper the duty of beneficence is the duty to do no harm (the duty of non-maleficence). It is obviously not beneficial overall to do something that in itself is beneficial if one wreaks havoc in the process, a danger to which modern doctors are particularly susceptible. Various medical obligations stem from the need to weigh the expected bad effects of any proposed intervention against the intended beneficial effects. The most obvious is the need to be good at one's job, and thus an effective medical education with continuous postgraduate updating can be seen to be a direct requirement of the principles of beneficence and non-maleficence.[3] Similarly, the content of that medical education needs constant scrutiny in the light of these principles. Audit[4] and clinical trials, not just for longevity but also for quality of life (including patients' own perceptions),[5][6] are obvious corollaries; it is essential properly to assess the types, amounts, and probabilities of benefit and harm that result or would result from one's clinical decisions.[7]

Respect for the patient's autonomy is needed once again, here as a component of non-maleficence, for people's conception of what they would find harmful is, like their conception of what they would find beneficial, intensely personal.[5][8] For example, one person will choose laryngectomy and a 60% three year survival rate for vocal cord cancer, whereas another will prefer radiation to spare his voice at the cost of a three year survival rate of only 30-40%.[9]

Another correlate of beneficence tempered by non-maleficence is effective, sympathetic, and adequate communication, for obviously in such delicate matters poor communication skills are likely to harm patients.[10][11] Incidentally, the ordinary, old fashioned medical virtues of friendliness, warmth, concern, and politeness (including good time keeping) remain obvious requirements of the principle of beneficence. It should hardly be worth stating except that my impression is that these seem to be decreasingly valued, especially in the public sector of British medical care. Can it be that a guaranteed income decreases concern within the profession for these beneficent attributes?

THE DUTY OF JUSTICE

Finally, beneficence must be tempered by justice. It seems clear and virtually beyond dispute that if all the available medical resources were used to provide care for only a favoured section of the sick population (say, the rich or members of a particular political party or race or just those whom the doctors fancied) no matter how beneficent and non-maleficent that care was, no matter how excellent, it would be unjustly, because unfairly, provided.

When medical resources are scarce (the inevitable case) some form of just distribution of those resources must be achieved. Such justice entails not only some form of fairness, of which more anon, but also efficiency in their provision. Here the growing business of cost benefit analysis and its variants is increasingly urged on the profession as a vital aspect of medical ethics.[12-16]

In this context doctors face a major dilemma. They may insist on raising their professional obligation to help their patients above the requirement of justice, arguing that it is not their business to share out inadequate resources but rather to do their best for the patients under their care[17][18] and to make as clear as possible the appalling results to other patients and potential patients of having inadequate resources. This position accords well with the circumscribed beneficence of the Hippocratic oath, which concentrates a doctor's moral obligation on "the benefit of my patients." Such doctors may see their position as similar to that of a barrister who does his utmost for his client and assumes that the other side will be equally partisan and that justice will result from such an adversarial system of advocacy. It is a reasonable approach provided that doctors accept the corollary that someone else (equivalent to the judge and jury) will decide, after listening to all their special pleading, on how the scarce medical resources are to be distributed most justly.

Alternatively, doctors may accept as part of their moral purpose not just the health of "my patients" but the health of all sick people, including future sick people (if medical research is to be justified) or, more broadly still (if preventive medicine is to be encompassed[19]), the health of all potentially sick people as part of their moral purpose. If they do so they clearly commit themselves and medical ethics to require justice in the distribution of medical resources: justice not only for their patients, not only for their country's patients, but for all the world's sick, present and future (and even perhaps the world's potentially sick).

Such a commitment if taken seriously would have quite staggeringly radical results in terms of taking away medical care from the well provided and redistributing it to the medically destitute. No wonder that we doctors have preferred to stick with the Hippocratic objective of concern for our patients. On the other hand, no wonder also that those concerned with fairness for all have sought—and continue to seek—to reduce medical control over the distribution of medical resources. It is a dilemma that the profession has on the whole evaded. If, however, we do not resolve it ourselves it is likely to be resolved for us.

References

1 Beauchamp TL, Childress JF. *Principles of biomedical ethics*. 2nd ed. Oxford: Oxford University Press, 1983:148-58.
2 Nozik R. *Anarchy, state, and utopia*. Oxford: Blackwell, 1974.
3 Crisp AH. Selection of medical students—is intelligence enough? *J R Soc Med* 1984;77:35-9.
4 McIntyre N, Popper K. The critical attitude in medicine: the need for a new ethics. *Br Med J* 1983;287:1919-23.
5 Greer S. Ethics of cancer treatment. *Soc Sci Med* 1984;18:345-9.
6 Rosser R, Kind P. A scale of valuations of states of illness: is there a social consensus? *Int J Epidemiol* 1978;7:347-58.
7 Wulff HR. *Rational diagnosis and treatment—an introduction to clinical decision-making*. 2nd ed. Oxford:Blackwell, 1981: especially 160-76.
8 Krupinski J. Health and quality of life. *Soc Sci Med* 1980;14A:203-11.
9 McNeil BJ, Weichselbaum R, Pauker SG. Speech and survival—tradeoffs between quality and quantity of life in laryngeal cancer. *N Engl J Med* 1981;305:982-7.

10 Anonymous. *Talking with patients—a teaching approach*. London: The Nuffield Provincial Hospitals Trust, 1979. (Note the useful annotated bibliography by C Fletcher.)
11 Pendleton D, Hasler J, eds. *Doctor-patient communication*. London: Academic Press, 1983.
12 Teeling Smith G, ed. *Measuring the social benefits of medicine*. London: Office of Health Economics, 1983.
13 Mooney GH. Medical ethics: an excuse for inefficiency? *J Med Ethics* 1984;**10**:183-5.
14 Mooney GH. Cost-benefit analysis and medical ethics. *J Med Ethics* 1980;**6**:177-9.
15 Kletz TA. Benefits and risks: their assessment in relation to human needs. *Endeavour* 1980;**4**:46-51.
16 Burchell A, Weeden R. Practical thoughts on cost-benefit analysis and health services. *Health Trends* 1982;**14**:56-60.
17 Levinsky NG. The doctor's master. *N Engl J Med* 1984;**311**:1573-5.
18 Parsons V, Lock P. Triage and the patient with renal failure. *J Med Ethics* 1980;**6**:173-6.
19 Owen D. Medicine, morality and the market. *Can Med Assoc J* 1984;**130**:1341-5.

Bibliography

A useful collection is Shelp EE, ed. *Beneficence and health care*. Dordrecht: Reidel, 1982. (See especially Buchanan's paper, Philosophical foundations of beneficence.)

CHAPTER 13

"Primum non nocere" and the principle of non-maleficence

Among the shibboleths of traditional medical ethics is the injunction "Primum non nocere"—first (or above all) do no harm. A recent textbook of psychiatric ethics calls it "the cardinal ethical principle sacred to medicine,"[1] and Veatch lists a representative collection of contemporary medical obeisances to this Latin tag.[2] While there is undoubtedly an important moral principle here, I shall argue that it does not have the simplicity, the absoluteness, or the priority that these words suggest.

No one seems to know the origins of the phrase "primum non nocere." It is not a literal translation of any part of the Hippocratic Oath, which requires doctors to do what they consider beneficial for their patients and to "abstain from whatever is deleterious and mischievous"[3]: nothing about "first" or "above all" do no harm there. Another possible source is a work in the Hippocratic corpus—the *Epidemics*.[4] However, the obscure literal translation of the relevant passage is simply: "To practise about diseases two: to help or not to harm"; and in the standard English translation Jones has "As to diseases make a habit of two things—to help, or, at least, to do no harm." A third possible source is a translation of the *Epidemics* by Galen, but he attached the "above all" to helping rather than to avoiding harm.[4] Thus the claim that avoiding doing harm must take priority in medical ethics does not even have the

80

authenticity of Hippocratic tradition—though even if it did, as I shall argue, it would be untenable.

Avoiding harm versus doing good

The claim that avoiding harm has priority over doing good is vigorously contested in moral philosophy. An interesting sample of the detailed arguments appears in a paper by Phillippa Foot in which she argues for the claim that "other things being equal, the obligation not to harm people is more stringent than the obligation to benefit people"[5] and in a detailed criticism of her paper by Nancy Davis,[6] who argues, primarily by counterexamples, that no such general priority can be defended. At first sight Foot's thesis is undoubtedly plausible. We seem to have what Kant called a perfect (though, many would add, only prima facie) duty to all other people not to harm them. On the other hand, we do not have a duty to benefit all other people; apart from everything else it is incoherent to talk of a duty which is impossible to fulfil. Thus at most we can have a duty only to benefit *some* other people (an imperfect duty), while we have a perfect duty to everybody not to harm them.

While it seems entirely plausible to claim that we owe non-maleficence, but not beneficence, to everybody, it does not follow from this that avoidance of doing harm (non-maleficence) takes priority over beneficence. All that follows is that the scope of non-maleficence is general, encompassing all other people, whereas the scope of beneficence is more specific, applying only to some people. Thus we can accept that each of us has a (prima facie) moral duty not to harm anybody else without being committed to believing that this prima facie duty must always take priority if it conflicts with any duty, including any duty of beneficence, we may have to particular people or groups of people.

No necessary priority for non-maleficence

The implausibility of the priority of non-maleficence can be shown by considering counterexamples. Medical practice often involves doing or risking harm to achieve a greater benefit for an individual—certainly the patients concerned would often vigorously contest a proposal that such risks should not be taken on the grounds that non-maleficence has moral priority over beneficence. (Equally, of course, in some cases they would consider the risk of harm to weigh heavier than the prospect of benefit.) At an interpersonal level vaccination programmes harm a few (those who suffer serious or fatal side effects) for the greater benefit of many. Driving motor cars harms some (the accident victims) for the benefit or at least pleasure of many. Taxation in proportion to means usually harms the taxed to benefit, among others, the sick, the hungry, and the poor—yet few would go along with Nozik[7] and claim that it was wrong to harm people by taxing them for these beneficial purposes.

Various ways of meeting such counterexamples to retain the principle that non-maleficence has moral priority over beneficence have been proposed. They include the doctrines of double effect, of the moral priority of acts over omissions, doings over allowings, negative over positive duties, and ordinary over extraordinary means. I shall return to some of these in subsequent chapters. Meanwhile suffice it to say that the claim that the general principle of non-maleficence necessarily has moral priority over any other moral principle, or even that it necessarily has priority over beneficence, cannot be sustained without considerable qualification; and many would argue that it cannot be sustained at all.

Therapeutic nihilism

In the case of medical ethics it is even more difficult to sustain, for in many clinical circumstances it simply makes no sense to separate beneficence and non-maleficence (some philosophers believe that it never makes sense to separate them and see non-maleficence as merely an aspect of beneficence.[8]) As the Hippocratic Oath says, the moral objectives in medicine are both beneficence—to help sick and suffering people—*and* to prevent harm in terms of both preventing deterioration of existing illness, damage, and disease and finding ways to prevent them in the first place. In both sorts of activity harm may be necessary to achieve benefit, risk of harm to achieve probability of benefit. A patient with a melanoma on her foot may have to lose a leg to save her life; a patient with Hodgkin's disease may have to undergo exceedingly unpleasant risks, including perhaps sterility, to have a reasonable chance of survival. Beneficence and non-maleficence in medical practice usually have to be considered and "weighed" together. If, however, the injunction "first (or above all) do no harm" were really to govern medicine such balancing would be prohibited and doctors would have to avoid intervening whenever there was a risk of harming their patients (or others)—which would be almost always. That way lies therapeutic nihilism, or minimalism, regardless of the potential benefits to be attained by risking more. Indeed, an American physician has suggested that it is just such a principle which guides the Federal Drugs Administration and prevents it from allowing American doctors to prescribe drugs which have been thoroughly investigated and accepted (despite their inevitable risks) in other countries.[9]

In inveighing thus against "primum non nocere" I am not opposing acceptance of the extremely important moral principle that one should avoid harming others. It is not, however, an absolute principle; it does not necessarily have priority in cases of conflict with other moral principles; and when there is also a moral obligation of beneficence the principle of non-maleficence has to be considered in that context. Similarly, and like the principle of beneficence itself, the principle of non-maleficence may conflict with the principles of respect for autonomy—for example, the patient may want to take bigger risks of harm in the pursuit of benefit than the physician would advise—and at least occasionally it may conflict with the principle of justice (the patient with Lassa fever may refuse to go to an isolation hospital, yet justice to others may override non-maleficence and require his compulsory isolation). All these complexities and qualifications are negated by the simplistic and apparently bogus formulation "primum non nocere": but stripped of this oversimplification the prima facie principle "non nocere" is a vital one for medical ethics.

Balancing risks and benefits

Perhaps its greatest importance is as a counterbalance to the doctor's primary special obligation to benefit his patients. Such benefit must always be assessed in the context of the risks and sometimes inevitabilities of harm which medical attempts to benefit so often entail. Moreover, just as I argued in the last chapter that benefit has to be assessed in the light of the principle of respect for autonomy, so too does harm. People's perception of harm, like their perception of benefit, is idiosyncratic, an integral part of the way they see themselves and of their life plan. One aspect of people's life plans is what the American lawyer Charles Fried calls their risk budget,[10] whereby people decide (however inchoately) the sorts of ends they wish to achieve and the sorts of risks—including risks of death—which they are prepared to take in pursuit of those ends. Although there are doubtless some general similarities, especially within fairly homogeneous societies, each person's risk budget is unique. Therefore it is important when applying the principle of non nocere to be aware of the individual's own assessment of what counts as harm. Once again this constraint on the principle of non-maleficence can be justified either on utilitarian grounds of maximising welfare or on Kantian grounds, in which respect for persons and their autonomy is the fundamental justification.

Albert Jonsen, an ex-Jesuit and a leading American medical ethicist (as they tongue twistingly insist on calling themselves), discerns several important moral strands entangled within the (sanitised) principle of non nocere. One reminds doctors that medicine is essentially a moral enterprise in which the infliction of harm, which is so frequently required in medical practice, can be justified only in the interests of "human benefit." (It is important here to distinguish between benefit to the patient—the primary special obligation of a doctor—and benefit to others, whether these be the patient's family, other patients, or people more generally.) A second strand reminds doctors that in assuming care they also assume an obligation to exercise "due care" (and once again such factors as an adequate medical training, regular postgraduate updating and audit can be seen as being required by the principle of non-maleficence). Two more strands remind doctors of the need to balance intended benefits against risks and inevitabilities of harm, physical, psychological, and social, as evaluated not only by the doctors but also by the patients and by society. Another strand reminds doctors of the problem that the Roman Catholic doctrine of double effect was designed to answer—notably, that one needs a way of assessing how to act when a proposed good action also has a risk or certainty of unintended but clearly foreseen bad effects. Finally, tentatively and "paradoxically" Jonsen suggests that sometimes it may be "legitimate to invoke the 'do no harm' maxim as a justification for termination of life"[4] (the context makes it clear that he is referring to withholding of treatment for the dying and irretrievably comatose).

Non-maleficence then is a crucial principle of medical ethics, though it usually needs to be considered in the context of coexisting obligations of beneficence and respect for autonomy and occasionally in the context of justice. "Primum non nocere," on the other hand, like, "The patient's interests always come first," is a phrase best consigned to the medical history books.

References

1 McGarry L, Chodoff P. The ethics of involuntary hospitalization. In: Bloch S, Chodoff P, eds. *Psychiatric ethics*. Oxford: Oxford University Press, 1981:217.
2 Veatch RM. *A theory of medical ethics*. New York: Basic Books, 1981:159-62, 344 (footnote 8).
3 British Medical Association. *The handbook of medical ethics*. London: BMA, 1984:69.
4 Jonsen AR. Do no harm: axiom of medical ethics. In: Spicker SF, Engelhardt HT, eds. *Philosophical medical ethics: its nature and significance*. Dordrecht: Reidel, 1977:27-41.
5 Foot P. The problem of abortion and the doctrine of double effect. Reprinted in: Steinbock B, ed. *Killing and letting die*. Englewood Cliffs: Prentice-Hall, 1980:156-65.
6 Davis N. The priority of avoiding harm. In: Steinbock B, ed. *Killing and letting die*. Englewood Cliffs: Prentice-Hall, 1980:172-214.
7 Nozik R. *Anarchy, state and utopia*. Oxford: Blackwell, 1974.
8 Frankena WK. *Ethics* (2nd ed). Englewood Cliffs: Prentice-Hall, 1973:45-8.
9 Gifford RW. "Primum non nocere." *JAMA* 1977;**238**:589-90.
10 Fried C. *An anatomy of values*. Cambridge, Massachusetts: Harvard University Press, 1970: 155-82.

CHAPTER 14

Justice and medical ethics

Some argue that medical ethics should have no truck with justice in the sense of fair adjudication between competing claims. Especially in the context of distributing scarce medical resources they take the view that the proper role of doctors is the Hippocratic one of doing the best they can for each patient. Their patients suffer when doctors start to temper this obligation with any conflicting considerations of fairness or justice.[1-4]

I pointed out in the chapter on beneficence that if doctors chose not to concern themselves with justice in medical practice then inevitably others would (and should) so concern themselves. In any case the idea that doctors can somehow legitimately evade any need to concern themselves with justice is hardly tenable given that in the course of their practice they are often confronted with conflicting claims on their resources, even from their own patients. The doctor who stays in theatre to finish a long and difficult operation and consequently misses an outpatient clinic is probably relying—implicitly or explicitly—on some sort of theory of justice whereby he can fairly decide to override his obligation to his outpatients in favour of his obligation to the patient on the table. So is the general practitioner who spends 30 minutes with the bereaved mother and only five with the lonely old lady who has a sore throat.

Nor do distributive concerns—the proper allocation of benefits and burdens—exhaust the relevance of justice to medical ethics. In the Arthur case the prosecution was concerned that those who break the law should be punished—an aspect of reparative, retributive, or corrective justice. Forensic psychiatrists, who concern themselves with the sanity or "competence" of clients charged with offences, are concerned with responsibility in the context of reparative justice. The Declaration of Tokyo's absolute prohibition of medical involvement in torture affirms a concept of justice based on rights that forbids certain things to be done to other people even if doing them may be of great social benefit. The General Medical Council, as a quasi court of law, is concerned with specifically legal aspects of justice. Even the selection of medical students or appointment of new medical colleagues (and the dismissal of old ones) requires justice. So the idea that justice is a moral issue that doctors can properly ignore is clearly mistaken.

Aristotle's principle of justice

Justice has always been one of the central concerns of philosophers, and indeed Aristotle's formal principle of justice is still widely accepted. Aristotle, somewhat hampered by the fact that the Greek word for justice was cognate with the Greek word for equality, was at pains to reject the claims of the democratic factions of Athens, who argued that justice meant equal shares for all (well, for all freemen). In a sophisticated treatment Aristotle distinguished between justice as another term for overall goodness or "complete virtue" and justice in a narrower sense, concerning equality of treatment. Such equality could not be sensibly understood as mere equal division of whatever benefit or burden was being considered, for "the origin of complaints and quarrels [is] when either equals have and are awarded unequal shares, or unequals equal shares."[5] Instead, argued Aristotle, the equality of justice had to be understood as meaning fair or proportionate treatment. He pointed out that in the latter sense justice was a relative term, in terms of relations both between people and for any one person between what he was owed and what he deserved. Those who deserved the same were owed the same, and in that sense justice required equality of treatment. Those, however, who deserved more were owed more, while those who deserved less were owed less. In both cases, as what they were owed was in strict proportion to their deserts, once again justice required people to be treated equally. The formal principle of justice or equality attributed to Aristotle is, therefore, that equals should be treated equally and unequals unequally in proportion to the relevant inequalities.[6]

The reason that Aristotle's formal principle remains so widely accepted is, of course, that it has little substantive content. It requires an equality of consideration (for an excellent contemporary analysis of the concept of equality see Bernard Williams's paper *The idea of equality*)[7]; fairness in the sense that conflicts are to be settled by mutually agreed principles of justice (for an account of fairness and fairplay see John Rawls's paper *Justice as fairness*)[8]; and impartiality in the sense that inequalities[9] of treatment cannot be arbitrary—based on mere opinion, preference, or partiality—but must be justified on the basis of, and in proportion to, relevant inequalities[9] (for a useful analysis of the concept of moral relevance see R M Hare's paper *Relevance*[10]). These concepts of fairness and impartiality, however, are also formal in that they do not specify the content of the "relevant inequalities" or the agreed principles. Different theories of justice can and do flesh out differently Aristotle's formal principle of justice with its demands for equal consideration, fairness, and impartiality. My somewhat contentious view is that these differences usually arise because priority is given to different moral principles as the basis for assessing people's just deserts. From the wide range of existing theories of justice five important types can be distinguished in this way.

Libertarian theories

Libertarian theories of justice emphasise that people should be accorded maximal respect for their personal liberty. Such theories usually start from a Lockean social contract designed to protect people's personal rights[11]—but, unlike Locke's theory, they often emphasise only the last of his natural rights to life, health, liberty, and possessions. The result is what might be called economic libertarianism, stemming from the theories of Adam Smith[12] via those of F A Hayek[13] (and in theory of the present governments of Mrs Thatcher and President Reagan) to that of the contemporary American philosopher Robert Nozik, who has purged these theories of any traces of utilitarian welfare maximising contaminants.

Although claiming to base his theory on a defence of Lockean natural rights, Nozik concentrates on only two of those rights; the right to life—that is, not to be unjustly killed—and the right to have possessions. Nozik argues that provided people acquire and transfer their "holdings" without violating others' rights no one is entitled to take them away. On that basis he argues that any taxation, beyond what is necessary to maintain the "minimal state" required to protect life and holdings, "is on a par with forced labour."[14]

Nozik's arguments have provoked vigorous philosophical response.[15] One of the criticisms is that if the whole spectrum of Lockean rights allegedly of concern to Nozik is to be protected his conclusions against taxation to benefit the poor and sick and otherwise disadvantaged are unsupported by his theory.

Utilitarian theories

Utilitarian theories emphasise that people deserve to have their welfare maximised. The danger of such theories is that in their simplistic versions they give too little weight to Lockean personal rights, which they are prepared to override whenever to do so is likely to maximise overall welfare. As I have indicated in my chapters on utilitarianism and autonomy sophisticated utilitarian theories from Mill onwards have shown awareness of these dangers and have incorporated moral concern for personal liberty (in the sense of autonomy) as a required condition of maximisation of welfare. Professor R M Hare's form of utilitarianism sees the formal principle of justice as "nothing but a restatement of the requirement that moral principles be universalisable"—a principle that according to Hare is manifested in Bentham's principle that everybody counts for one and nobody for more than one.[16]

Marxist theories

Marxist theories of justice emphasise that people deserve to have their needs met; people's "deserts" are thus in direct proportion to their needs and Aristotle's formal principle of justice can be met by making needs the relevant inequality. Apart from conceptual problems—what *are* needs?—Marxist moral theory faces objections similar to those levelled at simplistic utilitarianism—notably, that other moral concerns, particularly respect for individual autonomy, may be overriden in order to satisfy human needs. The Marxist corollary of "to each according to his needs" is "from each according to his ability," and the operation of this rule, according to Lenin, results in "actual equality."[17] It is a rule that, again in its

simplistic versions, brooks no rejection. ("The communists disdain
to conceal their views and aims. They openly declare that their ends
can be attained only by the forcible overthrow of all existing
conditions.")[18]

Once again we must distinguish between simplistic and sophisticated versions, for sophisticated Marxists are undoubtedly aware of
the dangers of inadequate concern for individual autonomy or
freedom,[19-21] and Marx himself sees a community of autonomous
people living together in peace, harmony, and true consciousness as
the utopian "objective" of the inexorable march of history.

Rawls's theory of justice

A highly influential attempt to blend utilitarian theories and those
theories of justice that respect autonomy—and indeed to incorporate the element of need of Marxist theories—is Professor John
Rawls's theory of justice.[22 23] As previously indicated, he argues that
people coming together to work out a theory of justice for their
society, and rendered impartial by the device of a "veil of ignorance"
whereby they do not know what role they are to have in that society,
would choose a system of justice whose first principle was that
people should have the maximal liberty compatible with the same
degree of liberty for everyone and whose second principle was that
deliberate inequalities were unjust unless they worked to the
advantage of the least well off.

Reward for merit

Finally, the claim that justice is essentially a matter of reward for
individual merit—the view, for instance, of W D Ross[24]—remains
plausible in at least some circumstances. For example, all competitions based on skill implicitly assume a principle of justice based
on merit, including competitions to enter medical schools or obtain
medical posts. Athletics competitions presuppose that "the best
man (or woman) wins." The structure of wages in a capitalist
society, whereby skilled work is rewarded more highly than
unskilled work, again presupposes both that skills confer merit and
that merit should be rewarded. On the other hand, can all
distribution of benefits and burdens be fairly or justly determined

on the basis of merit and demerit? In particular, there is no merit in being ill: should medical resources be allocated according to merit rather than illness?

So varied and so complex are theories of justice that more than with the other moral principles it would be hopeless even to suggest a generally acceptable substantive position. Instead it seems more useful to acknowledge that people's theories of justice are likely to continue to differ, I suspect largely on the basis of the relative weights they assign to the moral principles I have already outlined —that is, respect for autonomy, beneficence, and non-maleficence. I shall next look at allocation of scarce medical resources in the context of these various substantive theories of justice and in the light of Aristotle's formal principle of justice, which is implicitly accepted by them all.

References

1 Levinsky NG. The doctor's master. *N Engl J Med* 1984;**311**:1573-5.
2 Kemperman CJF. Clinical decisions. *Lancet* 1982;ii:1222.
3 Parsons V, Lock P. Triage and the patient with renal failure. *J Med Ethics* 1980;**6**:173-6.
4 Macara S, reported by Edwards S. No room for triage in NHS. *Medical News* 1983; 15-22 December:27.
5 Aristotle. *Nicomachean ethics*. 1131a:22-5.
6 Aristotle. *Nicomachean ethics*, Book 5 and *Politics*, Book 3, Chapter 9.
7 Williams B. The idea of equality. In: Williams B, ed. *Problems of the self*. Cambridge: Cambridge University Press, 1976:230-49.
8 Rawls J. Justice as fairness. *The Philosophical Review* 1958;**67**:164 94.
9 Benn S. Justice. In: Edwards P, ed. *The encyclopedia of philosophy*. New York, London: Collier Macmillan, 1967:298-302.
10 Hare RM. Relevance. In: Goldman AI, Kim J, eds. *Values and morals*. Dordrecht: Reidel, 1978:73-90.
11 Locke J. *Second treatise on government*. 1690. Chapter 2; section 6.
12 Smith A. *The wealth of nations*. 1776.
13 Hayek F. *Individualism and economic order*. Chicago: Chicago University Press, 1948.
14 Nozik R. *Anarchy, state, and utopia*. Oxford: Blackwell, 1974:169.
15 Paul J, ed. *Reading Nozik*. Oxford: Blackwell, 1981.
16 Hare RM. *Moral thinking: its levels, method and point*. Oxford: Clarendon Press, 1981:147-68.
17 Lenin VI. *The state and revolution*. Moscow: Progress Publishers, 1972:91.
18 Marx K, Engels F. Manifesto of the Communist Party. In: Hobsbawm EJ, ed. *The age of revolution*. London: Cardinal/Sphere, 1973:285.
19 Marcuse H. Freedom and the historical imperative. In: Marcuse H, ed. *Studies in critical philosophy*. London: Verso/NLB, 1972.
20 Kamenka E. *Marxism and ethics*. London: Macmillan, 1969.
21 Bottomore T, ed. *A dictionary of Marxist thought*. Oxford: Blackwell, 1985.
22 Rawls J. *A theory of justice*. Oxford: Oxford Univesity Press, 1976.
23 Daniels N, ed. *Reading Rawls*. Oxford: Blackwell, 1975.
24 Ross WD. *The right and the good*. Oxford: Clarendon Press, 1930:26-7.

Bibliography

Beauchamp TL. Justice. In: Beauchamp TL, ed. *Philosophical ethics: an introduction to moral philosophy*. New York: McGraw-Hill, 1982:219-58.

President's Commission for the study of ethical problems in medicine. *Securing access to health care*. Washington: US Government Printing Office, 1983.

Campbell AV. *Medicine, health and justice—the problem of priorities*. Edinburgh: Churchill Livingstone, 1978.

CHAPTER 15

Justice and allocation of medical resources

In the last chapter I indicated the wide range of issues concerning justice that are relevant to medical ethics. Even within the sphere of distributive justice the range is dauntingly broad. At one end of the range are what economists call microallocation decisions, of which the most dramatic deal with the allocation of scarce lifesaving resources such as haemodialysis between competing claimants. At the other end are macroallocation decisions taken at a governmental level on the division of the national "cake" between, for instance, health, other welfare, education, arts, and defence budgets. In between are varieties of what one might call mesoallocation decisions. These include decisions on how to distribute the allocated national health budget—the subject matter of the Black report,[1] which showed so clearly and so shockingly the statistical cor- relations throughout the nation between poverty and low social status on the one hand and adverse health outcomes on the other. (In doing so it also showed the inadequacy of assuming that overtly "health care" decisions are the only or even the most important ones in determining the nation's health.) They also include decisions on how to allocate medical resources at health authority level between the competing medical and other health care claims and decisions within a hospital on how to allocate between competing specialties and firms. More specific still are decisions for allocation among the different members of a hospital firm or health centre; and then come the microallocation decisions of each doctor or health worker distributing his or her available resources among particular patients. Although this range of decisions is exceedingly broad and disparate, all are based on some moral assessment of how competing claims can be fairly adjudicated. They are all thus explicitly or implicitly based on some theory of justice.

Preliminary distinctions

In the application of such a theory to problems of resource allocation it is worth making some preliminary distinctions. The first is between the formal and substantive contents of the theory. As I indicated in my last chapter, Aristotle's formal principle (equals should be treated equally, unequals unequally in proportion to the relevant inequality) and the impartiality and fairness it entails are widely accepted in different theories of justice whose substantive contents vary considerably. Among the substantive claims of a theory of justice (the function of which is fair adjudication between competing claims) it is important to distinguish its method for justifying itself and dealing with competing claims for other theories of justice (for we know that such conflicting claims are likely to occur). That method itself should meet Aristotle's formal requirements. A democratic voting structure, for example, affords a method of justly choosing between, among other things, the theories of justice preferred by different members of that democratic society. Finally, it is important to distinguish between the theory of justice itself and the equally important practicalities of applying it. Justice is not achieved simply by basing a scheme for resource allocation on a good theory of justice. Its decisions must be implemented.

Given the wide agreement about Aristotle's formal theory it is worth noting that its acceptance, even before any substantive aspects of a theory of justice are agreed, has important practical implications for resource allocation. Firstly, it requires resource allocation decisions to be made on moral grounds and it rules out partiality and other arbitrary methods of allocation. For instance, neither doctors nor governments can decide that they prefer blondes or whites and justly allocate their resources accordingly, because whiteness and blondness are not morally relevant characteristics (for a way of justifying this conclusion which purports not to depend on prior intuitive determination of moral principles see Hare's paper on relevance[2]). Secondly, in requiring fairness and thus an element of mutual agreement about the principles for settling conflicts Aristotle's formal principle seems (and this is an empirical not a logical claim) to require implementation of that legal adage that not only must justice be done it must also be seen to be done. People being as they are, only thus is such agreement likely to be obtained and maintained, and only thus are the agreed principles likely to be implemented consistently and impartially as formally required. Accepting this would have important practical implications for the way such decisions are taken.

Which moral principles should take precedence?

Once one turns to substantive theories of medical resource allocation—answers to the question "What are the relevant inequalities that justify giving more to some and less to others?"—one meets the same sort of disagreement and complexity about which moral principles should take precedence (see bibliography) as one does with theories of justice generally. The main alternatives, however, are straightforward enough, as my 8 year old daughter briskly reminded me when I was getting into my usual tangle over these impossible questions. How should I choose one out of three dying people to have the only available lifesaving machine?

"Well," she told me, sparing a minute or two from her television programme, "you could give it to the youngest because she'd live longer (welfare maximisation), or you could give it to the illest because she needs it most (medical need), or you could give it to the kindest because kind people deserve to be treated nicely (merit). No, you couldn't give it to the one you liked best (partiality), that wouldn't be fair." Nor, she decided, would "eenie meenie minee mo" (lottery) be fair because the one who needed it most, or the youngest, or the kindest might not get it. Nor did she (much to my surprise) think that the Queen should get it in preference to the poor man (social worth)—"because she's got so much already and the poor man hasn't." Of all the methods, her preferred one was to choose the illest because he needed it most—but, not surprisingly, she could not say why that was a better option than the others. Her list of options, however, is remarkably standard, and she joins many doctors in preferring medical need as the criterion of choice.

Perhaps unexpectedly medical need correlates most obviously with the Marxist criterion for justice—"to each according to his need." (I should add that this criterion is not exclusively Marxist, that few doctors are Marxists, and that few would accept the first half of the Marxist slogan—"From each according to his ability.") Unfortunately, the concept of a need—as distinct from a desire, for example—is not at all clear.[3] Furthermore, it is at least plausible to argue that assertion of needs entails assertion of implied value or values, in which case what are the implied values of the criterion of medical need? Prolongation of life, elimination of disease and attainment of health, and improved quality of life, in the sense of both reduction of suffering and enhancement of flourishing, are all candidates as values correlating to medical need but how are they to be chosen or ranked and what precisely do we mean by these terms? (Their complexities recall the World Health Organisation's definition of health as a state of complete physical, mental, and social wellbeing or the controversies over "sanctity of life," which I outlined in earlier chapters.) Thus the apparently straightforward criterion of medical need, while it is undoubtedly a necessary criterion for just distribution of medical resources,[4] in no way evades the need to make explicit the moral criteria it encompasses. Nor does it make any easier the choice between competing candidates agreed to be in medical need.

Medical success as a criterion

A related but by no means identical medical criterion is that of medical success. Medical resources should, it is often claimed, be allocated according to probability of medical success. This adds to the criterion of medical need one of efficiency and, like my daughter's criterion of maximal prolongation of life, corresponds roughly to the welfare maximising objective of utilitarian theories of justice. There are, of course, straightforward cases when the criterion is unproblematic: it would be absurd and wrong to give the only three available pints of a rare blood group to the patient with an incompatible group rather than to the patient with a compatible group. But the criterion of medical success is plagued by all the moral evaluative problems of medical need as well as by additional problems of how to determine medical success: what criteria are appropriate and how is success to be measured? (In this regard the economists' methods of comparing different techniques in terms of "quality adjusted life years" (QUALYs)[5] seem to offer conventional methods of clinical trial considerable additional precision for comparative purposes.)

The third plank of my daughter's analysis concerned merit and desert—save the life of the kindest because kind people deserve to be looked after. Other merit related criteria are forward looking rather than backward looking. A consultant physician would select "a man who would be able to continue regular work in suitable employment or a married woman with young children . . . in preference to an unemployed labourer with no fixed abode."[6] A consultant in clinical renal physiology, also writing about selection for renal dialysis, believed that "[g]ainful employment in a well chosen occupation is necessary to achieve the best results; only the minority wish to live on charity"[7] (even when the alternative is death?). More recently a man described as demented, intermittently violent, uncooperative, dirty, doubly incontinent, and with a tendency to expose himself and masturbate while being examined was taken off dialysis treatment "in the patient's best interests."[8] How much were the patient's dementia and discomfort the reason for stopping treatment and how much his objectionable behaviour?

How much, in general, should a patient's merits and demerits, personal and social, affect his being selected for livesaving medical treatment? Certainly in the medical triage of wartime return to combat duty has been an established medicomilitary criterion for treatment.[9] In peacetime, however, allocation of medical resources on the basis of a patient's non-medical merits is widely regarded as repugnant. How are we to account for such differing intuitions? And what about extreme cases such as Shackman's hypothetical choice between Fleming and Hitler, where only one of them could be treated?[10]

A possible approach

Given the fervent disagreement about which moral values should take priority in allocating medical resources it is hardly surprising that doctors on the whole tend to avoid the issue and try to concentrate on doing their best for their individual patients. Two methods of trying to cut the Gordian knot are notable. One commentator, in a different context, has argued that if not all who need scarce lifesaving resources can have them then none should.[11] Two American theologians, Ramsey and Childress, have argued that once a preliminary assessment on broad medical suitability has been made allocation should be by randomisation, either by a lottery or on a first come first served system (with steps taken to ensure that people could not unfairly "use" the system by having inside knowledge).[12][13]

I have not yet discovered an acceptable way to give consistent moral priority to any of these substantive criteria for allocation of scarce medical resources (and do not really expect to do so). Calabresi and Bobbitt plausibly suggest that societies tend to try to "limit the destructive impact of tragic choices between fundamental moral values by choosing to mix approaches over time."[14] Within such temporal cycles first one value and then another is emphasised, but "none can, for long, be abandoned." Be that as it may, it would be a mistake to suppose that either the possibility or the need for justice is undermined by such variability and disagreement about which fundamental moral value to abandon when, in a particular situation, not all can be retained. After all, justice is precisely a method for moral resolution of conflicting claims. Provided one or other fundamental moral value is given priority after due consideration of the different claims in the light of all of the agreed moral values and in accordance with the formal principle of justice then justice, it seems to me, is done.

Thus if, in the context of allocating scarce medical resources, practical systems were set up for resolving conflicts about which value, in a particular case, should have priority, and if those systems took account of the fundamental moral values of respect for autonomy, beneficence, and non-maleficence, and if their deliberative structures incorporated Aristotle's formal principle of justice with its demands of formal equity, impartiality, and fairness then they would be just systems and their deliberations could be expected to yield just results despite (perhaps because of) the conflict within them. I doubt if better than that is achievable. Is less acceptable?

References

1 Black DAK, Morris JN, Smith C, Townsend P, Davidson N. *Inequalities in health: the Black report.* Harmondsworth: Penguin, 1982.
2 Hare RM. Relevance. In: Goldman AI, Kim J, eds. *Values and morals.* Dordrecht: Reidel, 1978:73-90.

3 Daniels N. Health-care needs and distributive justice. *Philosophy and Public Affairs* 1981;**10(2)**: 146-79.
4 Williams B. The idea of equality. In: Williams B, ed. *Problems of the self.* Cambridge: Cambridge University Press, 1973:230-49.
5 Williams A. The economic role of "health indicators." In: Teeling-Smith G, ed. *Measuring the social benefits of medicine.* London: Office of Health Economics, 1983:63-7.
6 Nabarro JDN. Who best to make the choice? *Br Med J* 1967;i:622.
7 Parsons FM. A true "doctor's dilemma." *Br Med J* 1967;i:623.
8 Brahams D. When is discontinuation of dialysis justified? *Lancet* 1985;i:176-7.
9 Winslow GR. *Triage and justice.* Berkley: University of California Press, 1982:8.
10 Shackman R. Surgeon's point of view. *Br Med J* 1967;i:623-4.
11 Cahn E, cited by Calabresi G, Bobbitt P. *Tragic choices.* New York: Norton, 1978:188, 234.
12 Ramsey P. *The patient as person.* 10th ed. New Haven: Yale University Press, 1979:239-75 passim.
13 Childress J. Who shall live when not all can live? *Soundings: An Interdisciplinary Journal* 1970;**53(4)**:339–55. (Reprinted in: Gorovitz S, Macklin R, Jameton A, O'Connor J, Sherwin S, eds. *Moral problems in medicine.* 2nd ed. Englewood Cliffs: Prentice-Hall 1983:640-9.
14 Calabresi G, Bobbitt P. *Tragic choices.* New York: Norton, 1978:196.

Bibliography

(See also cited references)

Maxwell RJ. *Health and wealth.* Lexington: Lexington Books, 1981.
Boyd KM, ed. *The ethics of resource allocation.* Edinburgh: Edinburgh University Press, 1979.
Campbell A. *Medicine, health and justice—the problem of priorities.* Edinburgh: Churchill Livingstone, 1978.
Wolstenholme GEW, O'Connor M, eds. *Ethics in medical progress, with special reference to transplantation.* London: Churchill, 1966.
Childress J. *Priorities in biomedical ethics.* Philadelphia: Westminster Press, 1981.
Shelp E, ed. *Justice and health care.* Dordrecht: Reidel, 1980.
Engelhardt HT. Shattuck lecture: allocating scarce medical resources and the availability of organ transplantation. *N Engl J Med* 1984;**311**:66-71.
Rescher N. The allocation of exotic medical lifesaving therapy. *Ethics* 1969;**79(3)**:173-86.
Parsons V, Lock P. Triage and the patient with renal failure. *J Med Ethics* 1980;**6**:173-6.
Klein R. Rationing health care. *Br Med J* 1984;**289**:143-4.
Mooney G. Medical ethics: an excuse for inefficiency? *Journal of Medical Ethics*, 1984;**10**:183-5.

CHAPTER 16

Telling the truth and medical ethics

In this book I have discussed four principles for guiding action that seem to be required by any adequate philosophical theory of medical ethics: a principle of respect for persons, notably for their autonomy; a principle of beneficence; a principle of non-maleficence; and a principle of justice. Much moral debate stems either from disagreement about scope (about what sorts of entity are owed what sorts of moral concern) or from disagreement about the relative importance of these four principles. In the next four chapters I shall look at examples of conflicts in the context of medical ethics that are primarily between the principle of respect for autonomy on one hand and the principles of beneficence and non-maleficence on the other. I shall start with the issue of telling the truth.

Telling the truth

"In much wisdom is much grief: and he that increaseth knowledge increaseth sorrow"—(Ecclesiastes i, 18). Thus Dr Maurice Davidson began his chapter on truth telling in his 1957 book on medical ethics.[1] Davidson, however, argued against the tendency of "so many medical practitioners to withhold the facts from their patients, especially in cases of grave illness, and to insist that the truth must at all costs be kept from them." Rejecting this as a "fetich," which was wholly unjustifiable, he argued that real harm rarely resulted from honesty in response to patients who wanted reliable information about their condition. They might have "vitally important duties" that they could carry out only if they were given such information, and failure to divulge the plain facts was in the long run "a frequent cause of the greatest distress." As Davidson freely admitted, he was unusual among doctors in holding these views, but he remained unconvinced that the arguments of his colleagues against such frankness were "anything but an excuse for evading what is admittedly an extremely unpleasant duty."

Sympathetic as I am to Davidson's position, I think the opposing position needs more consideration. The case for deception in medical practice, whether in the context of fatal or grave disease or in informing patients of the risks of treatment or research, is usually based on three major arguments (elegantly dissected, among many others, by the philosopher Sissela Bok in her book *Lying*[2]).

The case for deception

The first argument in favour of deception is, as indicated above, that doctors' Hippocratic obligations to benefit and not harm their patients override any requirement of not deceiving people. For example, by definition patients with serious illness already have severe problems; the doctor adds to these problems by giving patients distressing news; moreover, patients' prospects of recovery often depend crucially on their morale and perhaps on some element of placebo effect or, in Balint's memorable phrase, "the drug doctor," or both. Passing on unpleasant medical information will probably undermine these and thus impair patients' prospects of recovery.

The second argument in favour of not telling the truth is that it cannot be communicated, both because a doctor is rarely, or never, in a position to know the truth (he can never be sure of the diagnosis or prognosis) and because even if he were the patient would rarely, if ever, be in a position to understand it. Even common words such as "cancer" are likely to be radically misunderstood by patients unless they have had a medical training. The wide range of conditions and prognoses and all other technical nuances implied by the word are probably not taken into consideration and are often replaced by a single dark understanding that cancer is simply another word for a peculiarly horrible death. As an American doctor emphatically summarised this argument, "It is meaningless to speak of telling the truth, the whole truth and nothing but the truth to a patient. It is meaningless because it is impossible" (he went on to recommend the "far older" medicomoral guide, "So far as possible do no harm").[3]

The third common medical argument against telling the truth is that patients do not wish to be told the truth when it is dire, particularly when they have a dangerous or fatal condition.

Precedence of beneficence and non-maleficence

With regard to the first argument—that the principles of beneficence and non-maleficence must take precedence over any requirement of not deceiving people—I showed in the chapter on autonomy how even for utilitarians (for whom the overriding moral principle is to maximise welfare and minimise harm) the principle of respect for autonomy is a crucial moral principle, while for Kantians respect for people and their autonomy is itself the overriding moral principle.

As deceiving people in medical contexts usually means failing to respect their autonomy (usually in each of the categories I outlined: thought, intention, and action) by denying them adequate information for rational deliberation, even from a utilitarian viewpoint it is probably morally unacceptable unless there is strong reason to believe that in a particular case overall welfare would be maximised by deception. Furthermore, the various arguments adduced in my discussion of medical paternalism apply to this specific example: not only can welfare be expected to be increased by honesty and frankness but also there is no reason to assume that doctors are particularly skilled judges of what course of action maximises welfare. Generally, so far as the welfare of individual patients is concerned they themselves are probably the best judges of whether knowing the truth about unpleasant facts will or will not improve their welfare.

There is, of course, an important practical difficulty here: how is the doctor to find out a patient's views without disclosing any unpleasant facts to those patients who would rather not know such information? There is no simple answer to this, but by sensitive questioning or by simply (but genuinely and at different times) offering to answer any questions, and giving adequate time for this, skilful doctors can often master this difficult medical art. In this context the remarkable psychological defence mechanism of denial may be reassuring; even after being told of their impending demise many patients seem to eliminate this information from their minds and deny that they have been given it, and, according to Kubler Ross, most people who know they are fatally ill tend to move in and out of such denial, more so to start with than later on.[4] Perhaps denial is a natural defence against being overburdened with such difficult thoughts when people are unable to cope with them. In addition to skilful and sympathetic discussion with patients after unpleasant information has been discovered, pilot studies could be run to find out the pros and cons of asking patients in advance their views on being deceived about unpleasant news, and indeed on a whole range of other medicomoral issues—an upgraded version of asking them what religion they espouse. For example, when they first registered with a doctor or attended a hospital patients could be offered an opportunity to answer a questionnaire about such matters, including how much they would like to participate in decision making or how much they would prefer to leave it to medical people; how much they would want to be told any bad news or how much they would wish to be shielded from it; whether or not they would wish to donate their organs if they died; whom they would allow to be told about their medical condition and whom not; which matters, if any, they considered to be particularly sensitive; and so on?

It astonishes me how, with a few exceptions, whenever I suggest this idea to medical colleagues there is widespread scorn—for example, "You'll terrify them," "What they say when they are fairly well couldn't be relied on when they are ill," "They might have changed their minds," "Suppose they have not understood the questions,"—yet when I suggest it to non-medical people the idea is usually embraced enthusiastically and the counterarguments rejected—"It might be worrying but at least the doctors would know what you wanted," "One wouldn't say something important unless one felt fairly sure about it," "Why shouldn't they design the questionnaire so that you did understand it?"

At the very least, it seems worth investigating such a scheme on a pilot basis to see if it offers any advantages in patient care and to find out what the problems are. Such an investigation would surely be as worthwhile for an MD thesis as many a more technical topic.

Impossibility of communicating the truth

The second argument against telling the truth concerns a fundamental confusion between the moral issue of truth telling and truthfulness on one hand and the epistemological, logical, and semantic problems that beset the concept of truth itself. Although these last three issues are of central importance in philosophy, they have little to do with the question of what it is right to do with such knowledge of the truth as a person believes himself to have. Here, the crucial moral issue concerns the doctor's intentions—in particular, does he intend to discover what the patient would wish to know and does he intend to try to meet such wishes when they concern the transmission of information that the doctor believes to be both true and likely to distress the patient, or does he intend to deceive the patient? Of course, most medical information is typically probabilistic, of course, patients will vary in their ability to understand complex medical information, of course, "the whole truth" is usually a mirage, and, of course, even philosophers disagree about what is meant by "truth." In the ordinary case none of these difficulties are relevant to the moral dilemmas of truthfulness and deceit. Those with residual doubts should, as Sissela Bok suggests,[2] imagine what their response would be to a used car dealer who used such arguments to justify his deceit.

Patients' wish not to know

Finally, there is the argument that patients do not want to be told the truth about their fatal condition. This is an important argument as it implicitly acknowledges that doctors ought to respect their patients' wishes. Several papers have, however, indicated that most people surveyed (usually over 80%) would like to be told the truth.[5-9] On the other hand, until fairly recently most American doctors surveyed generally withheld the truth about diagnoses of cancer from their patients,[10] though recently this has changed radically, with up to 97% of responding doctors preferring to tell patients with cancer their diagnosis.[11] Again this is an empirical question, but if the premise on which it is based is accepted—notably the desirability of doing what the patient wants—then the important issue is not what most patients or doctors think but what the particular patient in the particular circumstances wants. There seems to be no real doubt that the third argument is false and that at least some, possibly many, patients would wish to be dealt with honestly.

It should be emphasised that the forgoing counterarguments do not support indiscriminate, casual, curt, or unsupportive truth telling to all patients, approaches that are alas not unknown in medical practice, as Goldie disconcertingly recounts.[12] Nor do they deny the considerable difficulties concerned. They do reiterate that avoiding deceit is a basic moral norm, defensible from several moral perspectives, including those primarily concerned with maximising welfare, provided that welfare is not assessed simplistically on the basis of mere consideration of a patient's immediate distress on being told dire news.

References

1 Davidson M. What to tell the gravely ill patient, or one who has to undergo a serious operation. In: Davidson M, ed. *Medical ethics—a guide to students and practitioners*. London: Lloyd-Luke, 1957:109-19.

2 Bok S. *Lying—moral choice in public and private life*. Hassocks, Sussex: Harvester Press, 1978.

3 Henderson L. Physician and patient as a social system. *N Engl J Med* 1935;212:819-23.

4 Kubler-Ross E. *On death and dying*. London: Tavistock Publications 1970:34-43.

5 Cassem NH, Stewart RS. Management and care of the dying patient. *Int J Psychiatry Med* 1975;6:2-304.

6 Veatch r. *Death dying and the biological revolution*. New Haven and London: Yale University Press 1976:229-38.

7 Aitken-Swan J, Easson EC. Reactions of cancer patients on being told their diagnoses. *Br Med J* 1959;i:779-83.

8 McIntosh J. Patients' awareness and desire for information about diagnosed but undisclosed malignant disease. *Lancet* 1976;VII:300-3.

9 Kelly WD, Friesen SR. Do cancer patients want to be told? *Surgery* 1950;27:822-6.

10 Oken D. What to tell cancer patients. *JAMA* 1961;175:1120-8.

11 Novack DH, Plumer R, Smith RL, Ochitill H, Morrow GR, Bennett JM. Changes in physicians' attitudes toward telling the cancer patient. *JAMA* 1979;241:897-900.

12 Goldie L. The ethics of telling the patient. *J Med Ethics* 1982;8:128-33.

CHAPTER 17

Confidentiality

The principle of medical confidentiality—that doctors must keep their patients' secrets—is one of the most venerable moral obligations of medical ethics. The Hippocratic Oath enjoins: "Whatever, in connection with my professional practice, or not in connection with it, I see or hear, in the life of men, which ought not to be spoken of abroad, I will not divulge, as reckoning that all such should be kept secret."[1] The obligation is widely regarded as being exceedingly strict. Indeed, according to the World Medical Association's International Code of Medical Ethics it is an absolute requirement, even after the patient's death[2]: an absolutist claim echoed in a leading article in the *BMJ*.[3] (Ironically, two years later the General Medical Council (GMC) officially indicated to the editor of the *BMJ* that an obituary he had published of a famous soldier had transgressed medical confidentiality).[4] In France so strict is the obligation of medical confidentiality that it is apparently enshrined in law as an absolute medical privilege which no one, including the patient, is allowed to override, even when to do so would be in the patient's interest.[5]

In practice, on the other hand, doctors do not seem to regard confidentiality as an absolute requirement, as many relatives of seriously ill patients could testify. The BMA handbook of medical ethics lists five types of exception to the need to maintain medical confidentiality[6] and the GMC lists eight.[7] Recent British governments certainly do not regard medical confidentiality as absolute:

one of Mrs Thatcher's governments tried (unsuccessfully, largely as a result of opposition from the BMA) to give statutory licence to the police to search medical files,[8] and the BMA is still unhappy about the inadequate protection afforded to health records by the Data Protection Act 1984 and has cosponsored an interprofessional working group partly to tighten up the Act's provisions for medical confidentiality.[9] The campaign led by Mrs Gillick—accepted by the Court of Appeal but then rejected by the House of Lords—clearly believed that doctors are excessively concerned with confidentiality when it comes to prescribing oral contraceptives to girls under 16[10]; its members would presumably approve of the famous (or infamous) action of Dr Browne, who broke medical confidentiality and told his 16 year old patient's parents that she was taking the pill[11] (he was not censured by the GMC). Doctors express concern about both the threats to[12] and the relaxing standards of[13][14] the medical profession's principle of confidentiality, and one doctor has advocated that patients ought to keep their own records to preserve their confidentiality.[15] So was the American doctor right who called medical confidentiality "a decrepit concept"?[16] How can any sense be made of what may appear to be a chaotic jumble of attitudes?

What is "medical confidentiality"?

Some preliminary (and sketchy) analysis of the issues may be useful. What is meant by "medical confidentiality"? Is it morally valuable in itself or, if not, why is it morally important? Is it an absolute requirement? How does it relate to other obligations?

Essentially medical confidentiality is the respecting of other people's secrets (in the sense of information they do not wish to have further disclosed without their permission). There is obviously no general moral duty to respect other people's secrets (imagine a thief whom one had surprised saying "Shh, don't tell the police, it's a secret"), yet equally obviously doctors (and, of course, other groups) voluntarily undertake some general commitment to keep their patients' or clients' secrets (imagine the same thief talking about his activities in the course of a medical consultation). It seems clear that two conditions are necessary to create a moral duty of confidentiality: one person must undertake—that is, explicitly or implicitly promise—not to disclose another's secrets and that other person must disclose to the first person information that he considers to be secret. Thus there can be no transgression of confidentiality if the information is not regarded as secret by the person giving it; equally it is only because doctors have undertaken not to disclose patients' secrets that they have acquired a duty of confidentiality.

Why should doctors from the time of Hippocrates to the present have promised to keep their patients' secrets? If confidentiality is not a moral good in itself what moral good does it serve? The commonest justification for the duty of medical confidentiality is undoubtedly consequentialist: people's better health, welfare, the general good, and overall happiness are more likely to be attained if doctors are fully informed by their patients, and this is more likely if doctors undertake not to disclose their patients' secrets. Conversely, if patients did not believe that doctors would keep their secrets then either they would not divulge embarrassing but potentially medically important information, thus reducing their chances of getting the best medical care, or they would disclose such information and feel anxious and unhappy at the prospect of their secrets being made known.

Such consequentialist reasoning might well be accepted not only by utilitarians but also by many deontological pluralists. Deontologists, however, are unlikely to accept it as being adequate. They are likely to base their arguments for confidentiality not just (if at all) on welfare considerations but also on the moral principle of respect for autonomy[17] or sometimes on a putatively independent principle of respect for privacy,[18] which is seen as a fundamental moral requirement in itself.[19] [20] Thus, while the principle of medical confidentiality is not defended as a moral end in itself, it is defended by utilitarians and deontologists alike as a means to some morally desirable end—the general welfare, respect for people's autonomy, or respect for their privacy.

Medical confidentiality an "absolute" principle . . .

I have given reasons in previous chapters why both utilitarians and pluralist deontologists would not be able, and would not try, to make a principle such as medical confidentiality into an absolute principle, whereby a patient's confidences invariably had to be respected whatever the consequences (though the duty of confidentiality of the Roman Catholic confessor appears to be regarded as absolute). I have also argued previously that although the Kantian categorical imperative is regarded as an absolute principle, it necessarily requires the interests of all affected rational agents to be taken into account in its application; Kantians too would thus have no place for a maxim that demanded absolute medical confidentiality in all circumstances. Nor, incidentally, would there be any philosophical justification within these systems for the requirement of confidentiality to be absolute after a patient's death.

Such philosophical reluctance to see medical confidentiality as an absolute requirement is matched not only by various modern codes of medical ethics (though not by the World Medical Association's international code) but also, I suspect, by the Hippocratic Oath itself. The qualifier, "which ought not to be spoken of abroad," though ambiguous, can plausibly be taken to imply that the oath envisaged circumstances where it was permissible for information obtained in the course of a doctor's professional activities to be "spoken of abroad." In general the medical profession in Britain today probably sees confidentiality as a strong but by no means absolute moral obligation. The GMC's "blue book" lists the following eight legitimate exceptions: (a) when the patient "or his legal adviser" gives written and valid consent; (b) when other doctors or other health care professionals are participating in the patient's care; (c) when the doctor believes that a close relative or friend should know about the patient's health but it is medically undesirable to seek the patient's consent; (d) exceptionally when the doctor believes that disclosure to a third party other than a relative would be in the "best interests of the patient" and when the patient has rejected "every reasonable effort to persuade"; (e) when there are statutory requirements to disclose information; (f) when a judge or equivalent legal authority directs a doctor to disclose confidential medical information; (g) (rarely) when the public interest overrides the duty of confidentiality "such as for example investigation by the police of a grave or very serious crime"; and (h) for the purposes of medical research approved by a "recognised ethical committee."[7]

... or a "decrepit concept"?

Small wonder, the sceptic may be thinking, that Siegler called medical confidentiality a "decrepit concept." He had looked into the matter after a patient complained that all sorts of people whom he (the patient) had not authorised were looking at his notes. On investigation Dr Siegler was "astonished to learn that at least 25 and possibly as many as 100 health professionals and administrative personnel at our university hospital had access to the patient's record and that all of them had a legitimate need, indeed a professional responsibility, to open and use that chart." [16]

It is too harsh to call the principle of medical confidentiality "decrepit" but it does seem to have lost its way. The problem seems to be that the moral unacceptability of an absolute requirement of medical confidentiality has been recognised by the profession, which has both officially and in practice specified—without explicitly justifying—a set of ad hoc exceptions. On the other hand, doctors in practice (including myself I must confess) are reluctant to give up thinking and talking about confidentiality as though it were an absolute requirement. This reluctance may result partly from a lingering belief that it ought to be absolute and partly from the belief that if patients find out that it is not they will feel aggrieved, even betrayed, and also will stop being honest with their doctors, thus impairing their medical care. If my personal inquiries are representative few non-doctors are aware of how many official and de facto exceptions there are to medical confidentiality. On the other hand, many believe that the supposedly absolute requirement of confidentiality is actually honoured by doctors only in so far as it suits them. If these are typical attitudes doctors' current ambivalence about confidentiality is producing an understandable but undesirable cynicism about their attitudes.

Such cynicism could be reduced—without much if any harm to patient care—by admitting openly that medical confidentiality is not absolute and then justifying,[21] rather than simply stating, the sorts of exception approved by the profession, with a view to achieving a sort of "social contract" between the profession and society about the categories of exception that would and would not be acceptable. If such justification were attempted for each of the GMC's exceptions some would probably be more easily justifiable and more widely acceptable than others. Few people would expect doctors to undertake to disobey (just) laws or facilitate substantial and probable harm to others, yet those possibilities would be entailed by an absolute commitment to medical confidentiality, and it is presumably to combat such an unacceptable commitment that the GMC specified exceptions (e), (f), and (g).

Justification of exceptions

The other exceptions accepted by the GMC seem, however, less easily justifiable and less likely to obtain widespread social approval. Exception (*h*) justifies breaking confidentiality in order to carry out medical research—but ought not patients to be asked before their personal files are used for research? (This could be done routinely on admission or acceptance to a general practitioner's list and the files flagged appropriately.)

Exceptions (*b*), (*c*), and (*d*) are more problematical for they all depend on breaking a patient's confidence on the paternalistic assumption that to do so without consulting the patient will be in the patient's best interests. I have rehearsed the arguments against medical paternalism previously and they seem to be powerful (though I shall consider in a subsequent article certain exceptions such as emergencies, unobtainability of information about the patient's wishes, and mental incompetence or other causes of sufficiently impaired autonomy). In the normal case, however, I am persuaded that medical paternalism is an unjustifiable anachronism that would receive little if any support in any medicomoral "social contract" and which should be avoided. (Let me reiterate, however, that to object to paternalism is not to object to doctors making decisions if that is what the patient wants—the important thing is to find out what he or she does want.) Nor does there seem much reason to believe that obtaining a patient's consent to disclosure would be excessively difficult "at the sharp" end. ("Good morning Mrs Jones, I've been asked to give you physiotherapy, do you mind if I consult your notes to see what would be best for you?") Few patients are going to refuse what is in their own interests (especially if it is made clear that, as the GMC recommends, any health professional given access to the notes will be bound by the same strong though not absolute standards of confidentiality as are doctors). If patients do refuse certain others access to medical information about themselves, whether it is in the context of (*b*), (*c*), or (*d*), should not their refusal be honoured just as refusal to consult some other doctor or health professional would be honoured? Why not?

An important principle

In summary, medical confidentiality is an important medicomoral principle that can be justified by its contribution to improving people's medical treatment and respecting their autonomy and privacy. It is not, however, an absolute obligation, and this should be made clear. On the other hand, exceptions to medical confidentiality need to be not merely specified, as they are at present, but also justified. Exceptions based on the principles of non-maleficence and justice may well be justified in particular cases, but I have argued against accepting exceptions that are justified by appeals to medical paternalism or the benefits of medical research (both variants of the principle of beneficence which ignore its integral requirement also to respect people's autonomy). In both these sorts of cases patients' permission should generally be obtained if medical information concerning them is to be disclosed to others.

References

1 British Medical Association. *The handbook of medical ethics*. London: BMA, 1984:69-70.
2 British Medical Association. *The handbook of medical ethics*. London: BMA, 1984:70-2.
3 Parkes R. The duty of confidence. *Br Med J* 1982;285:1442-3.
4 Lock S. A question of confidence. *Br Med J* 1984;288:123-5.
5 Havard J. Medical confidence. *J Med Ethics* 1985;11:8-11.
6 British Medical Association. *The handbook of medical ethics*. London: BMA, 1984:12.
7 General Medical Council. *Professional conduct and disciplines: fitness to practise*. London: GMC, 1985:19-21.
8 Havard J. Doctors and the police. *Br Med J* 1983;286:742-3.
9 Macara AW. Confidentiality: a decrepit concept? *J R Soc Med* 1984;77:577-84.
10 Anonymous. Teenage confidence and consent. [Editorial.] *Br Med J* 1985;290:144-5.
11 Mason JK, McCall-Smith RA. *Law and medical ethics*. London: Butterworths, 1983:103.
12 Barnes J, Biggs S, Boyd R, *et al*. Threats to medical confidentiality. *Lancet* 1983;ii:1422.
13 Black D, Subotsky F. Medical ethics and child psychiatry. *J Med Ethics* 1982;8:5-8.
14 Pheby DFH. Changing practice on confidentiality: a cause for concern. *J Med Ethics* 1982;8:12-24.
15 Coleman V. Why patients should keep their records. *J Med Ethics* 1984;1:27-8.
16 Siegler M. Confidentiality in medicine: a decrepit concept. *New Engl J Med* 1982;307:1518-21.
17 Benn S. Privacy, freedom and respect for persons. In: Wasserstrom R, ed. *Today's moral problems*. New York: Macmillan, 1975:1-21.
18 Francis HWS. Gossips, eavesdroppers and peeping toms: a defence of the right of privacy. *J Med Ethics* 1982;8:134-43.
19 Caplan A. On privacy and confidentiality in social science research. In: Beauchamp TL, ed. *Ethical issues in social science research*. Baltimore: Johns Hopkins University Press, 1982:312-25.
20 Fried C. *An anatomy of values*. Cambridge, Massachusetts: Harvard University Press, 1970:137-52.
21 Sieghart P. Medical confidence, the law and computers. *J R Soc Med* 1984;77:656-62.

CHAPTER 18

Consent

Vets do not bother with their patients' consent: why should doctors? To address this question it is important to state which meaning of "consent" is being used for the term is ambiguous. Under one definition it simply means agreement, acceptance, or assent. It is fairly obvious (though here unargued) that this meaning of consent is not relevant to medical interventions, whether these are investigations, treatments, or research. For medical interventions it is widely accepted that consent means a voluntary, uncoerced decision, made by a sufficiently competent or autonomous person on the basis of adequate information and deliberation, to accept rather than reject some proposed course of action that will affect him or her.[1-14] Consent in this sense requires action by an autonomous agent based on adequate information and is by definition informed consent.

Autonomy and informed consent

This analysis explains why vets do not bother with consent from their patients: their patients are not autonomous agents (or at least most of them are not—I remain agnostic about certain higher primates and dolphins), and they simply could not give consent. Given that most adult patients could give consent in this sense, why should doctors bother to ensure that they do? The most obvious

113

answer is that generally we have a moral obligation to respect each other's autonomy, at least in so far as to do so is compatible with respect for the autonomy of others—a moral principle that I have previously shown to be supported from various moral perspectives. Doing things to other autonomous agents without their consent generally means overriding their autonomy. It is respect for people's autonomy, or self determination as Mason and McCall Smith[15] and Kirby[16] call it, that morally underpins the requirement of consent. Justice Kirby, then president of the Australian Law Reform Commission, in an excellent article on consent, wrote: "[T]he fundamental principle underlying consent is said to be a right of self determination: the principle or value choice of autonomy of the person . . . . The principle is not just a legal rule devised by one profession to harass another. It is an ethical principle which is simply reflected in legal rules because our law has been developed by judges sensitive to the practical application of generally held community ethical principles."[16]

According to the above definition, to consent to medical intervention a person requires sufficient information to be able to make an informed and deliberated choice, and it is in this context that doctors often object to the requirement for such consent. Patients, they say, are unnecessarily alarmed and their medical state unnecessarily impaired if they have to be given information about their diagnosis or prognosis or risks associated with their proposed management and treatment. The alarm is compounded with confusion, the argument continues, if differential diagnoses and risks have to be mentioned and made intolerable if the patient is expected to choose between the options. As Dr Ingelfinger exclaimed, he as a patient would not want "to be in the position of a shopper at the casbah who negotiates and haggles with the physician about what is best." Indeed, the doctor "who merely spreads an array of vendibles in front of the patient and then says 'go ahead and choose, it's your life' is guilty of shirking his duty, if not of malpractice."[17]

Three counterarguments

There are least three problems with such arguments. The first is that it is dangerous for a doctor to extrapolate from his own case to generalisations about his patients (or about anybody else). The fact that the good doctor would feel like that does not ensure or even make probable that any particular patient feels like that; and, as Dr Ingelfinger's argument implicitly acknowledges, the doctor should be trying to meet his patient's wishes rather than his own. As a wise philosopher once wrote, it is not putting yourself into another's shoes that is morally relevant, it is understanding what it is like for that other person to be in his or her own shoes that is morally important.

The second problem is empirical. Is it true that patients are generally made more alarmed by open minded and sympathetic provision of information and an invitation from the doctor to express their own preferences in so far as they have any? I doubt it. In this regard Dr Ingelfinger offers a parody of respect for the patient's autonomy when he suggests that the doctor would "haggle" with the patient or alternatively merely tell the patient the available options and then say "Go ahead and choose, it's your life." The doctor who really respected his patient's autonomy would discover in a sensitive way, which did not demand a particular answer, what and how much each patient really wanted to know and how much he wished to participate in the decision making. Some patients are, like Dr Ingelfinger, undoubtedly keen not to be given unpleasant information and to leave all the decision making to the doctor; if the doctor acts accordingly, thus respecting their autonomy, such patients will probably be happier. Other patients, however, do want to know about their medical condition and its implications and about alternative options; they also wish to be active in decision making when it affects them. Such patients will probably feel more at ease, trusting, and happy if the doctor has respected their wishes and if they have deliberately, comprehendingly, and willingly consented to their doctor's plan of management and have been "incorporated" as key figures in the medical management team. Of course, this second counterargument is no more than an empirical claim based on clinical impressions and common sense, but then so purports to be the claim it opposes—namely, that patients will be more miserable if they are given information they want and genuine opportunities to make their own decisions about their management.

The third problem is that even if it were true that in some circumstances a patient would be made more miserable by being given information about his condition and the risks of alternative methods of management, if that is what the patient truly wishes to know is the doctor not morally obliged to tell him? In the chapters on autonomy and paternalism I outlined what seem to me to be cogent arguments from utilitarian as well as deontological perspectives for respecting people's autonomy in so far as to do so is compatible with respecting the autonomy of others. These arguments have as much weight against witholding of relevant information required for consent as they do against lying or otherwise deceiving the patient (indeed the deliberate witholding of information relevant to decision making is a form of deceit) and against breaking confidentiality in the patient's own interests.

Doctors' licence under English law

A further set of common medical counterarguments to such emphasis on respect for patients' autonomy in the context of consent is that English law, at least with regard to consent to medical treatment, leaves doctors to decide, in the context of their therapeutic (as distinct from research) relationships, how much information they ought to give patients when obtaining their consent to treatment.

Accounts of what the law stipulates in any particular jurisdiction, however, do not in themselves provide moral justification for a moral claim. At most they can be used as part of a moral claim that there is a general presumption that it is a good thing to obey just laws. As I have argued previously, the possibility that there might be unjust laws (never mind the fact that there are) shows that it is not necessarily a good thing to obey all laws. Similarly, the possibility that there might be morally bad laws shows that what is legal is not necessarily morally justifiable.

The second point is that even if English law did leave it to doctors to decide how much information ought to be given to patients in the course of obtaining their consent to treatment doctors would still be obliged to try to resolve the moral problem: to be given the legal responsibility of making a moral decision is precisely not to be absolved from doing so.

It may, however, be worth noting that English law has recently been changed considerably by the House of Lords' appeal judgment in the Sidaway case.[18] Until that case the law seemed to leave decision making to doctors, although there is no legal unanimity about this.[19] Thus according to Lord Scarman's account of the relevant leading case, in which a Mr Bolam claimed, inter alia, that he had not been adequately informed about the risks of his (then unanaesthetised) electroconvulsive therapy, doctors would not be held negligent in law provided they acted "in accordance with the practice accepted by a responsible body of medical men," even if there existed a different practice advocated by another responsible body of doctors.[18] In the Sidaway judgment, however, only one of the five law lords (Lord Diplock) accepted the so called Bolam doctrine in its unmodified form. Each of the four others judged that the "professional standard" position of the Bolam doctrine required modification towards allowing patients to make their own decisions based on adequate information about treatments that included "material" (Scarman) or substantial (Bridge and Keith) risks, or "which might have disadvantages or dangers" (Templeman). Lords Bridge and Keith added that "When questioned by a patient of apparently sound mind about risks involved in a particular treatment proposed the doctor's duty was to answer both truthfully and as fully as the questioner required."[18]

Consent in therapeutic research

Occasionally the argument is heard that although properly informed consent is required in the context of non-therapeutic research on patients, it is not needed in the context of treatment or therapeutic research. The manifold medicomoral issues associated with medical research are complex but in this context suffice it to assert that doctors are no less morally obliged to respect the autonomy of their patients than that of their research subjects. The moral differences between the two categories relate not to respect for autonomy but to two quite different issues. The first is that there is a substantial danger that research subjects will assume that doctors' normal beneficent Hippocratic concern to do their best for their particular patients will also apply to their research subjects. In the case of non-therapeutic research this cannot be the case (by definition), and doctors therefore have a particularly strong moral obligation to make this clear to such subjects. The second, though related, point is that in the normal therapeutic relationship patients can properly assume that any risks to which the doctor proposes to subject them will be proposed only in the light of an analysis of risk and benefit that is favourable for the particular patient. Such an assumption would again be quite mistaken in the case of non-therapeutic research (in which the benefits, if any, will accrue to future patients, while the risks are taken by the research subjects). But while both these points indicate that doctors should make it crystal clear to patients when they are not acting in a therapeutic role, neither supports the claim that when doctors are acting therapeutically they need not obtain properly informed consent.

In the last three chapters I have argued that in normal cases respect for patients' autonomy takes moral priority over medical beneficence and generally precludes lying to or otherwise deceiving patients even in their own interests, breaking their confidences even in their own interests, and failing to obtain their adequately informed consent to medical intervention even in their own interests. In the next chapter I shall look at circumstances in which the principle of respect for autonomy does not seem to have priority over beneficence.

References

1 Wilkinson AW. Consent. In: Duncan AS, Dunstan GR, Welbourn RB, eds. *Dictionary of medical ethics*. London: Darton, Longman and Todd, 1981:113-7.
2 Taylor P. Consent, competency and ECT: a psychiatrist's view. *J Med Ethics* 1983;9:146-51.
3 Skegg PDG. Informed consent to medical procedures. *Med Sci Law* 1975;15:124-8.
4 Herbert V. Informed consent—a legal evaluation. *Cancer* 1980;46:1042-3.
5 Dunstan GR, Seller MJ, eds. *Consent in medicine*. London: King's Fund Publishing Office and Oxford University Press, 1983.
6 Beauchamp TL, Childress JF. *Principles of biomedical ethics*. 2nd ed. Oxford: Oxford University Press, 1983:69-93.
7 Lidz CW, Meisel A, Zerubavel E, Carter M, Sestak RM, Roth LH. *Informed consent*. London: Guilford Press, 1984.
8 Culver CM, Gert B. *Philosophy in medicine*. Oxford: Oxford University Press, 1982:42-63.
9 Gorovitz S. *Doctors' dilemmas*. London: Collier Macmillan, 1982:34-54.
10 Gorovitz S ed. *Moral problems in medicine*. 2nd ed. Englewood Cliffs: Prentice-Hall, 1983:153-91.
11 Reich WT, ed. *Encyclopedia of bioethics*. London: Collier Macmillan, 1978:751-78.
12 Levine RJ. *Ethics and regulation of clinical research*. Baltimore: Urban and Schwarzenberg, 1981:69-115.
13 Bankowski Z, Howard-Jones N, eds. *Human experimentation and medical ethics*. Geneva: Council for International Organisations of Medical Sciences, 1982:16-121.
14 Veatch RM. *Case studies in medical ethics*. Cambridge, Massachusetts: Harvard University Press, 1977:290-316.
15 Mason JK, Smith RAM. *Law and medical ethics*. London: Butterworths, 1983:120.
16 Kirby MD. Informed consent: what does it mean? *J Med Ethics* 1983;9:69-75.
17 Ingelfinger FJ. Arrogance. *N Engl J Med* 1980;303:1507-11.
18 Anonymous. Sidaway v Bethlem Royal Hospital and the Maudsley Hospital Health Authority and others (law report). *The Times* 1985 Feb 22:28.
19 Norrie K McK. Medical negligence: who sets the standard? *J Med Ethics* 1985;11:135-7.

CHAPTER 19

Where respect for autonomy is not the answer

In several of the chapters in this book I have emphasised the centrality of the principle of respect for autonomy to many areas of medical ethics, as indeed to ethics in general, and I have shown how this centrality is a feature of both utilitarian and deontological theories of ethics. Undoubtedly, doctors will have thought of counterexample after counterexample deriving from their clinical practice when respect for autonomy does not seem to be the most important or relevant moral principal. In this chapter I shall outline several categories of clinical circumstances in which, so I shall argue, respect for autonomy is not the central moral issue. They include examples in which patients have given prior consent for their doctors to make decisions on their behalf; in which respect for the autonomy of a particular patient conflicts with respect for the autonomy of others or causes harm to others or conflicts with considerations of justice; in which the patient has either no autonomy or too little autonomy for the principle of respect for autonomy to apply; and of emergencies in which it is not possible to find out what the patient himself would wish to happen.

I have already discussed the fact that often patients positively and deliberately delegate doctors to make decisions and manage their case. Provided the patients have made an autonomous choice then the doctor who accedes to their request and makes the decisions is indeed respecting their autonomy. In these circumstances the Hippocratic principles of medical beneficence and non-maleficence to the patient are the main moral determinants, though, as I have argued, they may have to be constrained by considerations of justice. Let me recall that the principle of respect for autonomy—whether in the utilitarian model of Mill or in the deontological model of Kant—has built into it the need to consider the autonomy of others: a point too often forgotten by overenthusiastic libertarians. I have also argued against any moral principle being taken as absolute—the principle of respect for autonomy may conflict with the principles of beneficence, non-maleficence, and justice (though I have also argued from both deontological and utilitarian standpoints that where others will not be harmed such conflicts usually require respect for the patient's autonomy).

Impaired autonomy

The most obvious counterexamples to the primacy of respect for autonomy arise either when the patient has no autonomy—for example, a baby has no autonomy—or, more difficult still, when patients have considerably impaired or otherwise inadequate autonomy—for example, when they are young and immature or severely mentally handicapped or disordered, from whatever cause. One of the complicating features of medical practice is that disease and disability tend precisely to impair people's autonomy to a greater or lesser extent.[123] The crucial question then arises, How much autonomy does a person need to have for his autonomy to require respect?

It is perhaps worth distinguishing between impairments of the three types of autonomy I discussed in my chapter on autonomy: of action, of will (or intention), and of thought. Impairment of autonomy of action, however gross, does not in itself justify overriding the principle of respect for autonomy. This becomes immediately obvious if severely physically handicapped people are considered; their impaired autonomy of action in no way reduces our moral obligation to respect their autonomy of thought and of will, though respect for their autonomy must as usual be balanced against respect for the autonomy of others. Physically handicapped people, especially those needing wheelchairs, often complain, however, that they are treated as though their autonomy is generally impaired and typically as though they are children ("Does he take sugar?").

When autonomy of thought or will, or both, are sufficiently impaired medical intervention without consent that will benefit the person concerned—that is, paternalistic intervention—often seems to be justified, and indeed morally imperative, even when the person concerned rejects such help. A child with meningitis should surely be given her antibiotic injections even if she hates injections and volubly refuses them; a severely mentally handicapped adult should surely be operated on for appendicitis even if he does not want an operation. The most plausible justification for overriding such decisions is that (*a*) it is in the patient's best interests to do so and (*b*) such patients do not have sufficient autonomy of thought for their self damaging decisions to require the respect due to autonomous agents (though, as the American president's commission on medical ethics concluded in a useful report, this should in no way stop doctors from consulting such people and, as far as is consistent with their best interests, acceding to their opinions and preferences[4]).

Impaired autonomy of thought is not necessarily a matter of impaired reasoning; reasoning may be fairly unimpaired but based on an information substrate that is grossly distorted by, for example, delusions, false perceptions, hallucinations, or a mixture. Even that apostle of non-paternalism, J S Mill, argued that paternalistic interference was justified to benefit the mad or delirious, children, and the immature and that in general "those who are still in a state to require being taken care of by others must be protected against their own actions as well as against external injury."[5]

Impaired volitional autonomy

Not only may autonomy of thought, including reasoning and cognition, be grossly impaired but so too can volitional autonomy—that is, impaired autonomy of will or intention (a point approached from a different perspective in an excellent analysis of these issues by Professors C M Culver and B Gert, one a psychiatrist, the other a philosopher[6]). Such impairment of volition may be intrinsic or extrinsic. The case of extrinsic impairment raises the interesting issue of duress. Clearly, an agreement to participate in some clinical trial would hardly be voluntary if the "volunteer" and his family were threatened with death if he refused. But what about an offer of payment? Most of our decisions are subject to some degree of external pressure. At one end of the spectrum such pressures are clearly powerful enough grossly to impair our autonomy of will or intention; at the other end they are equally clearly within the normal range of "pros and cons," consideration of which necessarily plays a part in voluntary choice.

Similarly, the mere presence of intrinsic pressures such as stress, neurosis, and grief, although they may diminish a person's autonomy, does not justify overriding what is left. On the other hand, gross intrinsic impairment of volitional autonomy may also occur and is especially obvious in certain psychiatric conditions, including severe depression and certain phobias. Dr Pamela Taylor, in a symposium on putatively "irrational" yet "competently made" decisions to refuse electroconvulsive therapy, graphically recalls that some psychiatric patients are simply not able to make voluntary decisions of any kind.[7] As well as psychiatric illnesses various severe "physical" illnesses and toxic agents can cause grossly impaired autonomy of will (alcohol and barbiturates are used by seducers and interrogators for precisely this purpose). When people's autonomy of volition is sufficiently diminished by such impediments, though not when it is merely diminished,[8] then the autonomy that remains may justifiably be overridden not only if it threatens others but also if it threatens them.

Such examples from psychiatric practice are entirely consistent with the obvious claims that: (*a*) autonomy is not an all or nothing affair and (*b*) a basic minimum of autonomy is required for the principle of respect for autonomy to be applicable. They do not alas give answers to the major question that I started with, How much autonomy is "sufficient" for a person to be respected as an autonomous agent? Nor do they answer the questions, Who is to decide how much autonomy a particular person possesses and on what basis, and Who is to make decisions (such as giving or withholding consent by proxy to medical intervention) on behalf of those judged non-autonomous or "incompetent," and according to what criteria?

I can do no more than outline a few points here in the context of these important questions. Although there are no clear cut answers to the question of how much autonomy a person must have to have it respected, it appears reasonable to argue that at least in democratic, and hence in principle autonomy respecting, societies there seems no good reason for doctors to establish any higher (or lower) standards of requisite autonomy than those set democratically. In our society these standards are not high, and little autonomy is required to be allowed by law to make legally valid contracts, marry, consent to sexual intercourse, vote, make a will, go motor racing, hang gliding, horse riding, and mountaineering, join the army, drive and motor cycle, smoke, drink alcohol, and generally participate in risk taking and risk inflicting occupations and in general take responsibility for one's own decisions. It seems reasonable for doctors, unless they are required by the democratic process to do otherwise, to accept that people possessing similarly minimal standards of autonomy should none the less have that autonomy respected in the context of medical care (in so far as such respect is compatible with respect for the autonomy of others).

Dialogue between the profession and society

This seems pre-eminently an area in which far more dialogue is needed between the profession and society. It may be that were non-professionals to have a better awareness of the depredations of severe disease, both physical and mental, on a person's autonomy of thought or will, or both, they would wish to raise the threshold required for autonomy to be respected. People in our society might agree with those like Professor J F Drane who proposes that required standards of "competence" to make decisions on medical care for oneself should vary with the seriousness of those decisions. Thus to be respected as competent to make decisions that are "very dangerous and run counter to both professional and public rationality"—for example, a decision to refuse lifesaving treatment —would require a far higher standard of manifest competence to make informed, voluntary, deliberated, and thus autonomous decisions than would less dangerous decisions, including a decision to accept the same treatment.[9 10]

Dialogue between the profession and society seems necessary to decide on the two other problems mentioned: who should decide how much autonomy a person possesses, and on what criteria, and who should make decisions by proxy, and by what criteria, for those patients classified as inadequately autonomous or incompetent? Reasonable arguments could be offered for those with special training, such as forensic psychiatrists and psychologists, to make the assessments of patients' autonomy, and doing so in relation to the particular decisions that need to be made; reports on methodology abound.[6][11-15]

Similarly, reasonable arguments can be offered in favour of people previously designated by the patient, or their next of kin or other loved ones being proxies for inadequately autonomous patients (except in emergencies where delay would be dangerous), these proxies having an option to delegate part or all of their proxy decision making to doctors if they believe this to be in the patient's interests. I would, however, agree with Professor Kennedy that such proposals are not the prerogative of doctors to implement without social agreement.[16] After all, it is fairly uncontroversial to assert that the source of any authority or rights that we as a profession have to make decisions about other people's medical care, notably the source of our right to be beneficent to any patient, is either that person's own autonomous desire that we do so or something simplistically but most easily summarised as "the will of society." In cases where the patient does not have such an autonomous desire, including a previously expressed prospective desire,[17] it follows that the source of our authority to behave paternalistically towards him must be society. Hence our obligation to lay the ground rules for such beneficent medical paternalism in consultation with that society of which we form a part.

References

1 Pellegrino ED. Toward a reconstruction of medical morality: the primacy of the act of profession and the fact of illness. *J Med Philos* 1979;4:32-56.
2 Freud A. The doctor-patient relationship. In: Gorovitz S, ed. *Moral problems in medicine.* 2nd ed. Englewood Cliffs, London: Prentice-Hall, 1983:108-10.
3 Perry C. Paternalism as a supererogatory act. Cited by: Jones GE. The doctor-patient relationship and euthanasia. *J Med Ethics* 1982;8:195-8.
4 President's Commission for the Study of Ethical Problems in Medicine and Biomedical and Behavioural Research. *Making health care decisions.* Washington: US Government Printing Office, 1982:181.
5 Mill JS. On liberty. In: Warnock M, ed. *Utilitarianism.* 11th ed. Glasgow: Collins/Fontana, 1974:135-6,229.
6 Culver CM, Gert B. *Philosophy in medicine.* Oxford, New York: Oxford University Press, 1982:109-25. (See also chapters 3, 7, 8.)
7 Taylor PJ. Consent, competency and ECT: a psychiatrist's view. *J Med Ethics* 1983;9:146-51.
8 Anonymous. Impaired autonomy and rejection of treatment [Editorial]. *J Med Ethics* 1983;9: 131- 2.
9 Drane JF. *The many faces of competency. Hastings Center Report* 1985;15:17-21.
10 Eth S. Competency and consent to treatment. *JAMA* 1985;253:778-9.

11 Bloch S, Chodoff P, eds. *Psychiatric ethics*. Oxford, New York: Oxford University Press, 1981:203-94.

12 Edwards RB, ed. *Psychiatry and ethics*. Buffalo: Prometheus Books, 1982:68-82,189-346,496-605.

13 Roth LH, Meisel A, Lidz CW. Tests of competency to consent to treatment. *Am J Psychiatry* 1977;**134**:279-84.

14 Roth LH, Lidz CW, Meisel A, *et al*. Competency to decide about treatment or research: an overview of some empirical data. *Int J Law Psychiatry* 1982;5:29-50.

15 Bluglass R. *A guide to the Mental Health Act 1983*. Edinburgh: Churchill Livingstone, 1983:75-88.

16 Kennedy I. *The unmasking of medicine*. London: George Allen and Unwin, 1981:76-98.

17 Robertson GS. Dealing with the brain damaged old—dignity before sanctity. *J Med Ethics* 1982;**8**:173-9.

CHAPTER 20

Acts and omissions, killing and letting die

One of the central arguments in the moral defence of Dr Arthur was that, although it was impermissible for a doctor to kill his patient, it was sometimes morally permissible to allow the patient to die and that such permissibility extended to cases of newborn infants with severe handicaps. Whether this distinction between killing and letting die is thought to be morally relevant in cases of newborn infants with Down's syndrome rejected by their parents (the case confronted by Dr Arthur), few doctors doubt its relevance to *some* medicomoral problems. Such cases include patients with fatal diseases who would actually prefer to be dead. Although some doctors would be prepared to espouse voluntary euthanasia and kill these patients,[1] most, like the BMA's *Handbook of Medical Ethics*,[2] would probably reject killing yet be prepared to withhold lifesaving treatment knowing that the omission would probably result in an earlier death than would be the case if treatment were given.[3]

The distinction is often referred to in the context of euthanasia by the satiric lines of Arthur Clough, now raised by many in the medical profession to near holy writ: "Thou shalt not kill but needs't not strive officiously to keep alive."[4] What, if any, moral importance resides in the distinction between killing and letting die?

126

Acts and omissions doctrine

One argument is that actions that result in some undesirable consequence are always morally worse than inactions, or failures to act, that have the same consequence—an argument that I call the acts and omissions doctrine. Intuitively, such a doctrine seems attractive, and indeed some would say obviously true. If I do not send a cheque to Oxfam someone will probably die who otherwise would not have died. Suppose I discover who that person is and send him (in addition to my cheque to Oxfam) a small personal food parcel containing a Danish pastry that I have carefully flavoured with the appropriate almond flavoured poison. Would I then have a moral defence that as there is no morally relevant difference between acts and omissions I was doing nothing worse in sending the poisoned cake than if I had not sent the cheque to Oxfam?[5]

Of course, in that example, it is worse to kill the person, and any moral theory that could not justify this conclusion would stand condemned by that fact alone by an argument of reductio ad absurdum. However, it is not the acts and omissions doctrine that explains the moral distinction.

Of the many philosophical attacks against the acts and omissions doctrine, perhaps one of the simplest is shown in the imaginary counterexample offered by Rachels.[6] Starting from a consideration of the famous "Johns Hopkins case," in which on parental request an infant with Down's syndrome with duodenal atresia was not operated on and died[7]—a case whose mirror image was the English case "re B," in which in similar circumstances a court ruled that the infant had to be operated on[8]—Rachels offers a "philosopher's example" to show that the bare distinction between acts and omissions is not necessarily morally important. Smith and Jones both stand to inherit fortunes if their 6 year old cousins predecease them. Smith drowns his cousin in the bath, making it seem like an accident. Jones intends to drown his cousin but on creeping into the bathroom sees the boy slip, bang his head, and slide unconscious beneath the water. Jones waits to make sure that the boy really does die and is ready to push his head back under the water if he should surface, but the boy drowns accidentally.

The two cases are almost identical except that one is a case of an act and the other of an omission. Yet, argues Rachels, no one would want to argue that there was any moral difference between the two cases; in particular, no one would argue that Jones was any less morally culpable than Smith. Rachels concludes therefore that in the absence of other morally important differences the bare distinction between acts and omissions, between killing and letting die, is not itself morally relevant.

It is, of course, no use retreating to the position that sometimes acts with a given consequence are worse than omissions with that consequence unless you can also say what it is that makes the moral difference; whatever that something is it must be different from the bare difference between acts and omissions.

Moral difference between killing and letting die

Sometimes the difference is seen as one of harming versus benefiting: whereas a doctor has a responsibility not to harm his patient, it may be claimed that he is not obliged always to help the patient. Although this may be a plausible defence for people who do not have particular obligations to help patients, being a doctor includes voluntarily undertaking an obligation to help one's patients—that, indeed, is the primary purpose of medicine. Thus it would be absurd for a doctor to try to justify an omission to provide lifesaving treatment for his patient on the grounds that he had no moral obligation to help his patient.

Can it be that the intuitive moral difference between cases of killing and letting die is really based on overall considerations of harm and benefit to the patient and that in cases in which doctors feel justified in not providing lifesaving treatment the justification is really that to do so would not benefit the patient (and probably harm him)? Undoubtedly, such assessments of harm and benefit are essential for all medical interventions, but again they are not equivalent to the acts and omissions doctrine, as an example should make clear. A patient suffering from untreatable widespread metastatic cancer has been labelled by the consultant and his ward team as "Do not resuscitate"; cardiopulmonary resuscitation would not, they think, benefit him and would probably harm him. The patient has a myocardial infarction in the presence of the consultant, who quite deliberately does not resuscitate him, and the patient dies. This is a case of an omission—a letting die—that the consultant considers justifiable as he believes that overall the patient would not have benefited from the omitted action.

Now consider the same patient except that this time the houseman and cardiac arrest team on night duty have resuscitated him after his infarction, and he is unconscious on a respirator, the heart having been restarted successfully. The consultant still believes that cardiopulmonary resuscitation would not benefit this patient; indeed, he is more certain than ever for there is some evidence that the resuscitation was not started until several minutes after the arrest and there is probably additional anoxic brain damage. The consultant turns off and disconnects the respirator, and the patient dies almost immediately. There is no doubt that the consultant has acted in the second case, as distinct from omitting to act in the first, and has caused the death of the patient (assuming he was not already brain dead).

If this causal account of the matter is still resisted the reader should ask whether the consultant who did the same thing for bad motives—for example, to get away for the weekend—would be described as causing the patient's death by disconnecting the ventilator. According to common medical interpretation of the Clough doctrine, the consultant's omission was morally correct in the first case, but his action in the second case was morally unacceptable. If, on the other hand, the moral analysis is based on an assessment of overall harms and benefits to the patient then if the omission in the first case is morally acceptable so too must be the action in the second case; in fact in the second case there will be better reason to believe that the patient would not have benefited by continuing life support. Clearly, assessment of harm and benefit to the patient is not equivalent to deciding whether it is the doctor's action or omission that has led to the patient's death—that is, deciding whether killing or letting die has occurred.

Rejection of doctrine by Roman Catholics

The acts and omissions doctrine outlined above is sometimes thought to be a Roman Catholic doctrine, but it is no such thing; as vigorous a rejection of this doctrine is offered by Roman Catholic philosophers and theologians[9][10] as by secular philosophers,[6][11][12] and one reason for its recent explicit rejection by Roman Catholics concerned with medical ethics is the way that doctors have used it to defend actions such as Dr Arthur's.[13]

Crucial to the Roman Catholic rejection of the simple, indeed simplistic, acts and omissions doctrine in relation to killing and letting die are several moral claims. Firstly, an omission by definition is not simply any inaction but a morally culpable inaction. Thus there must be some additional moral information given before any particular inaction can be classified as an omission, for, as Aquinas first defined it, "Omission means failing to do good, albeit not any good but only the good that one ought to do."[9] On this account it is absurd to talk about omissions being morally acceptable because, by definition, all omissions are morally unacceptable.

The second moral claim made by the Roman Catholics is that not only does outcome matter when a moral judgment is made on a person's action but so too do preceding considerations, including pre-existing moral obligations and the understanding and intention with which the person acted. Few sophisticated moral philosophers would disagree with that; although simplistic utilitarians (usually non-philosophers) sometimes deny it, it would be mistaken to suppose that this represents a moral gulf separating Roman Catholic or other deontologists from utilitarians.

The philosophy of action is a complicated and contentious subject,[14] but there is little doubt that both the consequences of an action and the agent's beliefs and intentions about what he is doing are relevant to its moral assessment. Here Roman Catholic theology has sought to differentiate between intended and unintended consequences of an action, notably in the principle of double effect. I shall consider some problems associated with this principle in the next chapter, but the claim that we can justifiably differentiate betweeen those consequences of our actions and inactions that we intend, those that we foresee but do not intend, and those that we do not intend or foresee at all seems important though complex.

The third Roman Catholic moral claim in this context is that certain sorts of action and inaction are absolutely forbidden; in particular, intentional killing of an innocent person, including bringing about death by omission, is absolutely forbidden. On the other hand, intentional actions and omissions not intended to bring about death but as a result of which death may be foreseen may in some circumstances be morally permissible. There are problems with such distinctions between foreseeing and intending to which I shall return, and I have already indicated the morally paralysing effect of pluralist absolutism, acceptance of which entails the logical impossibility of acting rightly in circumstances in which moral absolutes conflict. Moreover, to many of us there seem to be such intuitively obvious counterexamples: during the Falklands war a soldier was reported to have shot his trapped comrade in response to his comrade's anguished pleas that he was burning to death in a situation from which there was no possibility of saving him. Was that morally wrong?

Of course, all moral thinkers would agree that the injunction against intentionally bringing about the death of innocent subjects is of central importance to all societies and that it should be inculcated as a very strong rule of moral life. To claim, however, that it is an absolute principle never to be transgressed, irrespective of the strength of other morally valid reasons favouring such transgression in a particular case, is to many of us utterly implausible in the light of real and theoretical counterexamples. Surely moral life is just more complicated than such simple absolutism suggests,[15] though, of course, the opposite position is also widespread and fervently supported.[16]

References

1 Brewer C. Let our patients die. *BMA News Review* 1985;11:16.
2 British Medical Association. *Handbook of medical ethics.* London: British Medical Association, 1984:64-5.
3 Bayliss RIS. Thou shalt not strive officiously. *Br Med J* 1982;285:1373-5.
4 Clough AH. The latest decalogue. Cited in Glover J. *Causing death and saving lives.* Harmondsworth: Penguin, 1977:92.
5 Foot P. The problem of abortion and the doctrine of the double effect. Reprinted in: Steinbock B, ed. *Killing and letting die.* Englewood Cliffs: Prentice-Hall, 1980:156-65.
6 Rachels J. Active and passive euthanasia. *N Engl J Med* 1975;292:78-80. Reprinted in Steinbock.[5]
7 Gustafson JM. Mongolism, parental desires, and the right to life. *Perspect Biol Med* 1973;16: 529-59.
8 Mason JK, McCall Smith RA. *Law and medical ethics.* London: Butterworths, 1983:84-5.
9 Linacre Centre. *Prolongation of life, paper 2. Is there a morally significant difference between killing and letting die?* London: Linacre Centre, 1978.
10 Mahoney J. *Bioethics and belief.* London: Sheed and Ward, 1984:36-51.
11 Glover J. *Causing death and saving lives.* Harmondsworth: Penguin, 1977:92-116.
12 Harris J. *The value of life.* London: Routledge and Kegan Paul, 1985:28-47.
13 Linacre Centre. *Euthanasia and clinical practice: trends, principles and alternatives.* London: Linacre Centre, 1984.
14 White AR, ed. *The philosophy of action.* Oxford: Oxford University Press, 1968. (A useful introductory collection of papers; see also Anscombe GEM. *Intention.* Oxford: Blackwell, 1957.)
15 Bennett J. Morality and consequences. In: McMurrin M, ed. *The Tanner lectures on human values, 1981.* Cambridge: Cambridge University Press, 1981:45-116.
16 Casey J. Actions and consequences. In: Casey J, ed. *Morality and moral reasoning.* London: Methuen, 1971:155-205.

Bibliography

There is a vast range of relevant papers as the subject is important in the treatment of newborn handicapped infants; intensive care; cardiopulmonary resuscitation; the application or withholding of medical and surgical resources in life threatening conditions whether for purposes of rationing or reasons of benevolence; treatment of the elderly and the senile; treatment of the terminally ill; treatment of the permanently unconscious; and the concept and management of brain stem death. A small selection follows:

President's Commission for the Study of Ethical Problems in Medicine. *Deciding to forgo life sustaining treatment*. Washington: US Government Printing Office, 1983.

Beauchamp TL, Childress JF. *Principles of biomedical ethics*. 2nd ed. Oxford, New York: Oxford University Press, 1983:106-47.

Gorovitz S, Macklin R, Jameton A, O'Connor J, Sherwin S, eds. *Moral problems in medicine*. 2nd ed. Englewood Cliffs: Prentice-Hall, 1983.

Campbell AGM, Duff RS. Deciding the care of severely malformed or dying infants. *J Med Ethics* 1979;5:65-7.

Sherlock R. Selective non-treatment of newborns (a reply to the previous reference with a further response from A G M Campbell and R S Duff). *J Med Ethics* 1979;5:139-42.

Harris J. Ethical problems in the management of some severely handicapped children (with commentaries by J Lorber, G E M Anscombe, and D J Cusine). *J Med Ethics* 1981;7:117-24.

Shearer A. *Everybody's ethics: what future for handicapped babies?* London: Campaign for Mentally Handicapped People, 1984.

Murray TH. The final, anticlimactic rule on baby Doe. *Hastings Cent Rep* 1985;15(suppl 3):5-9.

Jennett B. Inappropriate use of intensive care. *Br Med J* 1984;289:1709-11.

Miles SH, Cranford R, Schultz AL. The do-not-resuscitate order in a teaching hospital: considerations and a suggested policy. *Ann Intern Med* 1982;96:660-4.

Lo B, Steinbrook RL. Deciding whether to resuscitate. *Arch Intern Med* 1983;143(suppl 8):1561-3.

Lynn J, Childress JF. Must patients always be given food and water? *Hastings Cent Rep* 1983;13(suppl 5):17-21.

Pallis C. Whole-brain death reconsidered—physiological facts and philosophy. *J Med Ethics* 1983;9:32-7.

CHAPTER 21

The principle of double effect and medical ethics

In the last chapter I argued that there was no morally relevant difference between acts as a class and omissions as a class, and, in particular, between that subclass of actions described as killings and that subclass of omissions described as allowing to die. Does that mean that the widespread and deeply held intuition—widespread within law, medicine, and religion—that there is a morally important distinction here should simply be rejected? Does it mean that Clough's couplet: "Thou shalt not kill; but needs't not strive officiously to keep alive" should be regarded as no more than the satiric piece of nonsense he probably intended it to be? Strictly speaking I think the answer is yes; but two more or less related moral distinctions, while they do not support the acts and omissions doctrine, do support a rule of thumb, no more, that often corresponds with Clough's couplet. Both distinctions are reflected in important Roman Catholic moral doctrines—ordinary and extraordinary means, which I shall look at in the next chapter, and double effect, which I analyse here. Both doctrines, which Roman Catholic doctors are likely to have studied in considerably greater depth elsewhere,[1-8] are of general interest in philosophical medical ethics.

133

Evil in the pursuit of good

The doctrine of double effect was developed in its earliest form by Aquinas to delineate the conditions in which it is morally legitimate to cause or permit evil in the pursuit of good. One of its central distinctions is between the intentional causation of evil—for example, intentionally bringing about another person's death (whether by action or omission)—and foreseeing evil (including another's death) to be a consequence, either inevitably or probably, of what one does or omits to do. While I shall argue that the full doctrine is not ultimately defensible, unless one also accepts its absolutist theological presuppositions, and is indeed vigorously criticised even from within the Roman Catholic faith,[12] it is an early and admirable attempt to confront the complexity of moral decision making in contexts when intended good effects of actions are inevitably or probably going to be accompanied by unintended but foreseeable bad effects.

Perhaps the most important general reminder for medical ethics that emerges from the doctrine of double effect is that actions cannot be morally judged solely in terms of their consequences. The conditions under which they are carried out, including the intention with which they are carried out, is a vital aspect of their moral assessment.[9] If I shoot a peasant in the woods thinking that his brightly plumed hat is a pheasant then, while the consequences of my shooting are as bad as they would have been had I intended to murder him, none the less, my action of shooting with intent to kill a pheasant is morally better than my action of shooting with intent to murder a peasant would be. This is but a tiny example of the complexity of the notion of human action (a useful introduction to which is given in White's collection of philosophical readings[10]), but it illustrates the crucial moral importance of intention.

It also reminds us of the difficulties of finding out what the real facts of the matter may have been ("Of course, m'lud, I was not trying to do away with the old lady so as to get my hands on her bequest. I was just trying to save her from suffering"). Such (epistemic) difficulties in finding out the facts are quite different from questions about what those facts actually are and questions concerning moral evaluation of those facts. Thus although it is difficult to be certain what a person's intention in acting actually was, we none the less try to do so because it makes a difference to our moral evaluation of his action.

Distinctions between moral evaluations

In this context the distinctions alluded to earlier are important: between moral evaluation of the state of affairs that results from a person's action, moral evaluation of the action independently of its results, and moral evaluation of the agent himself. A person may have a fundamentally good or bad character and yet take specific actions that are atypical of his character, and the results of any of these particular actions may be bad despite the action being good or good despite the action being bad. Thus a thoroughly nasty surgeon (bad character) may take thoroughly admirable action in performing a difficult operation to try to save the life of his otherwise severely disabled patient (good action) and yet kill the patient on the table (bad result).

Given all that preliminary sorting, let us look at what the doctrine of double effect actually says. It states, in the context of actions that have both good and bad effects, that: doing an action that has a bad effect is permissible if (*a*) the action is good in itself, (*b*) the intention is solely to produce the good effect, (*c*) the good effect is not achieved through the bad effect, and (*d*) there is sufficient reason to permit the bad effect.[11]

Only the fourth of those clauses is fairly uncontroversial (and widely accepted as vitally important to philosophical medical ethics). It requires that a bad effect may be risked or brought about only if there is "sufficient" (or, as some writers put it, "proportionately grave"[2]) reason to do so. In other words, there may be justification for bringing about or risking evil but only if the good expected is sufficiently weighty to overcome the usual prohibition against doing so. Of course, the clause raises a host of associated issues, including the problem of how one balances goods and evils against one another and the important and under-investigated issues of risk and medical ethics.[12-14]

Clearly, in deciding whether a bad effect is justified in the pursuit of a good effect not only must the relevant "weights" of each be assessed but also their respective probabilities. The lower the probability of their occurrence the more both harms and benefits must be discounted. There is no substantial doubt, however, that it may be entirely legitimate to take an action to try to achieve some good end—for example, the saving of a patient's life threatened by a malignant melanoma on his foot—even when one knows that this can be achieved only at the cost of some certain harms, such as the amputation of his leg (admittedly a medically controversial assumption), and others that are more or less probable, such as postoperative pain, phantom foot experiences, the adverse effects of chemotherapy and radiotherapy, death from anaesthetic, postoperative pulmonary embolus, and so on. Conversely, it would be morally naive to look at some medical action in retrospect, see that its results were in fact disastrous, such as the patient's dying, and conclude that therefore the action must have been wrong.

Must an action be "good in itself"?

The first three components of the doctrine of double effect are essentially reflections of the moral absolutism of standard Roman Catholic morality and so can be expected not to appeal to those who reject such absolutism. None the less, each has important lessons even for the non-absolutist. The first implies that unless the proposed action, shorn of its consequences, is good or at least morally neutral then it is morally unacceptable. But suppose a doctor believes, for example, that unless he lies to a patient about the death of his entire family in a car crash (the patient himself being critically ill and under intensive care) there would be a substantial risk that his anguish would kill the patient. Many of us would find such lying more or less repugnant but justified as part of the morally more important enterprise of keeping the patient alive over his acute critical phase. The good achieved would for many of us be a sufficient or proportionately grave reason to justify the evil of lying during that critical phase. And if this example is unconvincing, what about lying to the Gestapo about the presence of the fugitive allied soldier or Jew or resistance fighter in one's cellar? Yet the first clause of the doctrine of double effect should rule out, in principle, such life-saving lying. Thus for non-absolutists the first clause is too demanding; but it does importantly remind us that one's proposed action may in itself be morally unacceptable quite apart from its consequences. If so the pluralist would seek to "weigh" the evil intrinsic to the proposed action against other moral considerations including any good that it would be likely to achieve, as required in the fourth clause. The difficulties of such weighing, to which I have repeatedly alluded, will seem to the pluralist less morally objectionable than the counterintuitive results of absolutism.

Intention solely to produce the good effect?

The second clause requires that "the intention is solely to produce the good effect." There are at least two problems with this. The first is that when one knows that a bad effect will result from one's action then it seems to be simply self deceiving, perhaps hypocritical, to say that one does not intend it. Imagine a surgeon saying that he does not intend the patient's loss of a leg as he puts him on the list for an amputation, that he merely foresees that result, that his intention is only to save the patient from dying from disseminated cancer. The second problem is that even when it is only probable that an unintended bad effect will occur—for example, that a patient will become sterile from cytotoxic chemotherapy—there remains a general assumption that as moral agents we should accept moral responsibility for effects we foreseeingly cause, even though we do not intend them. Most would go further and say we should accept moral responsibility for effects the risks of which we ought to have foreseen, even if we have not foreseen them. If these assumptions are accepted then we cannot get off the moral hook simply by saying, however truthfully, that, although we foresaw the probability of a certain bad result, we did not intend that result, only the good result.[15]

What analysis of this clause of the principle of double effect does seem to show is that for a careful moral evaluation of an action or proposed action it is important to distinguish between (a) the intended end and the intended means to that end; (b) the intended results, whether means or ends, of one's actions and the unintended but foreseen risks of side effects of one's action; (c) the desired results and intended results—doctors and their patients repeatedly intend, as means to some desirable result, certain undesirable results; and (d) the overall result, all things considered, of one's proposed action and the individual components of that overall result. For each of these distinctions it seems possible to suggest morally plausible medical examples in which one component is bad, the other good, and in which provided one can reasonably expect to achieve a balance of good over evil and provided that that balance meets the "proportionality" requirements of the crucial fourth clause of the principle, then the proposed action would be justifiable.

Justification of good ends by bad means

The third clause of the doctrine, according to which the good effect must not be achieved by means of the bad effect is again likely to be rejected by non-absolutists as counterintuitive on the grounds that sometimes it *is* justifiable to achieve a good end by a bad means. The case of the amputation above seems an obvious example, though perhaps every surgical operation affords one. Thus to be deprived of a leg is obviously a horrible effect of the decision to amputate; but if removal of that leg is the least damaging way of securing a reasonable chance of saving a patient's life, and assuming that that is what the patient wants, then few would reject such treatment, given the magnitude of the benefit predicted, despite the fact that the good effect can be achieved only by means of the bad effect, thus transgressing this third clause of the doctrine of double effect. (Heroic redescriptions of the amputation to avoid this conflict are frankly unconvincing.) The conflict between good and bad effects would be assessed by those who rejected this clause by appeal, once again, to the requirement of proportionality or sufficient reason in the fourth clause.

In summary then, while the doctrine of double effect points up some important facts about the nature of moral judgment, including the need, when judging the morality of actions, to take the agent's intentions into account, it is unlikely to be accepted in full by non-absolutists (and is indeed rejected by many Roman Catholics). What remains virtually unassailed are its claims (*a*) that evil can rightly be done or even risked only in the pursuit of doing good and (*b*) that evil may rightly be done or even risked only if there is sufficiently weighty (or proportionately grave) reason to justify it. As doctors acquire ever more dangerous and unpleasant techniques in their unremitting quest to benefit their patients these residual components of the doctrine of double effect crucially serve both to justify and to restrict their application.

References

1 Curran CE. Roman Catholicism. In: Reich WT, ed. *Encyclopedia of bioethics*. London, New York: Collier Macmillan, 1978:1522-34.
2 May WE. Double effect. In: Reich WT, ed. *Encyclopedia of bioethics*. London, New York: Collier Macmillan, 1978:316-20.
3 Linacre Centre. *Prolongation of life. I. The principle of respect for human life*. London: Linacre Centre, 1978.

4 Linacre Centre. *Prolongation of life. II. Is there a morally significant difference between killing and letting die?* London: Linacre Centre, 1978.

5 Linacre Centre. *Prolongation of life. III. Ordinary and extraordinary means of prolonging life.* London: Linacre Centre, 1979.

6 Working Party. *Euthanasia and clinical practice—trends principles and alternatives.* London: Linacre Centre, 1982. (Report.)

7 Mahoney J. *Bioethics and belief.* London: Sheed and Ward, 1984.

8 Grisez G, Boyle JM. *Life and death with liberty and justice—a contribution to the euthanasia debate.* Paris, London: University of Notre Dame Press, 1979.

9 Anscombe GEM. *Intention.* Oxford: Blackwell, 1957.

10 White AR, ed. *The philosophy of action.* Oxford: Oxford University Press, 1968.

11 Linacre Centre. *Prolongation of life. I. The principle of respect for human life.* London: Linacre Centre, 1978:10.

12 Pochin E. Risk and medical ethics. *J Med Ethics* 1982;8:180-4.

13 Anonymous. Risk [Editorial]. *J Med Ethics* 1982;8:171-2.

14 Childress JF. Risk. In: Reich WT, ed. *Encyclopedia of bioethics.* London, New York: Collier Macmillan, 1978:1516-22.

15 President's commission for the study of ethical problems in medicine. *Deciding to forego life sustaining treatment.* Washington: US Government Printing Office, 1983:77-82.

Bibliography

Foot P. The problem of abortion and the doctrine of double effect. In: Steinbock B, ed. *Killing and letting die.* Englewood Cliffs: Prentice-Hall, 1980:156-65.

Locke D. The choice between lives. *Philosophy* 1982;57:453-75.

CHAPTER 22

Ordinary and extraordinary means

In the last two chapters I pursued the theme of killing versus letting die, and particularly the "Clough doctrine": thou shalt not kill; but needs't not strive officiously to keep alive. I argued that no consistent moral difference could be found between acts and omissions to support the Clough doctrine but that something similar could be supported as a rule of thumb by accepting that intentionally bringing about the death of one's patients (whether by action or omission) is, at least generally speaking, wrong (I argued against the absolutist claim that it is without exception wrong). On the other hand, knowingly risking death or other harm in the pursuit of the patient's good may often be justified, provided the importance of the good and its probability of being attained are sufficiently great to outweigh that risk of death or other harm. This position corresponds, at least roughly, with the fourth clause of the Roman Catholic doctrine of double effect.

In this chapter I wish to pursue the same theme, and especially the question of striving to keep alive, via another Roman Catholic doctrine, that of ordinary and extraordinary means. Unravelled and stripped of its misleading name, this doctrine offers patients and doctors, regardless of their religious orientation, a reasonable and straightforward basis for assessing how much to strive to keep alive. To this critical non-Catholic the doctrine seems remarkably similar to the fourth clause of the doctrine of double effect, which again seemed uncontroversial in requiring sufficient or proportionately grave reason when the pursuit of good means risking or inflicting harm. Thus the doctrine of ordinary and extraordinary means states, in essence, that the good of saving life is morally obligatory only if its pursuit is not excessively burdensome or disproportionate in relation to the expected benefits.

The distinction between ordinary and extraordinary means seems to have been introduced in Roman Catholic theology in the sixteenth century by the Spanish theologian Dominic Banez, who said that while it was reasonable to require people to conserve their lives by ordinary means such as ordinary nourishment, clothing, and medicine, even at the cost of ordinary pain or suffering, people were not morally required to inflict on themselves extraordinary pain or anguish or undertakings that were disproportionate to their state in life.[1] The doctrine was applied by Pope Pius XII in 1957 to an anaesthetist's questions about when to use and stop using mechanical respirators in the case of deeply unconscious patients, who, if not already dead, would be likely to die soon after disconnection from mechanical ventilation.[2,3] According to the Pope, people had "the right and the duty in case of serious illness to take the necessary treatment for the preservation of life and health." "Normally," however, "one is held to use only ordinary means— according to circumstances of persons, places, times, and cultures —that is to say means that do not involve any grave burden for oneself or another. A more strict obligation would be too burdensome for most men and would render the attainment of the higher more important good too difficult. Life, health, all temporal activities are in fact subordinated to spiritual ends."

Doctors can act only with patient's permission

In relation to the doctor's obligations the Pope reminded his audience of anaesthetists that "the rights and duties of the doctor are correlative to those of the patient. The doctor in fact has no separate or independent right where the patient is concerned. In general he can take action only if the patient explicitly or implicitly, directly or indirectly gives him permission." So far as the techniques of resuscitation in such circumstances are concerned patients and doctors are morally permitted to use them, but since they "go

beyond the ordinary means to which one is bound, it cannot be held
that there is an obligation to use them, nor consequently that one is
bound to give the doctor permission to use them." Families too
must base their decisions in such matters on the "presumed will of
the unconscious patient if he is of age and 'sui juris.' Where the
proper and independent duty of the family is concerned they are
usually bound only to the use of ordinary means. Consequently if it
appears that the attempt at resuscitation constitutes in reality such a
burden for the family that one cannot in all conscience impose it
upon them, they can lawfully insist that the doctor should
discontinue these attempts and the doctor can lawfully comply."[3]
(The Pope went on to state that such compliance was not euthanasia
in the sense of intentionally bringing about a patient's death, for it
was never more than an indirect cause of the cessation of life, and he
justified this assertion by appealing to the principle of double effect
and the distinction between causation—namely, of the ensuing
death—for which a person is morally responsible—"voluntarium in
causa"—and that for which he is not responsible.) The contents of
this papal allocution have been widely accepted within the Roman
Catholic faith and were reaffirmed in the 1980 Declaration on
Euthanasia of the Sacred Congregation for the Doctrine of the
Faith.[4]

"Circumstances of persons, places, times, and cultures"

What becomes immediately clear from these various complex
accounts is that the doctrine of ordinary and extraordinary means is
not simply a matter of looking at some proposed treatment, asking
whether it is ordinary or extraordinary in the usual dictionary sense
of the terms—that is, common or uncommon, usual or unusual,
mundane or exceptional—and then concluding that if the treatment
is ordinary it is morally obligatory, if extraordinary it is morally
optional. There is no question, therefore, of looking for some
morally neutral description of the proposed treatment (Is it common
rather than uncommon, simple rather than complicated, non-
technological rather than technological, and so on?) and deriving
from that a moral conclusion. As usual, one cannot derive an
"ought" from an "is"[5] (a morally neutral is, that is). Instead, as these
accounts and various contemporary accounts emphasise,[6-10] the
proposed treatment has to be assessed on the basis of what would be

excessively or disproportionately burdensome in the context of the particular patient in his particular circumstances—as Pope Pius XII put it, in the context of "circumstances of persons, places, times, and cultures—that is to say means that do not entail any grave burden for oneself or another." Only after the assessment of whether the burden of treatment would be too great for, or disproportionate to, the likely benefit in the particular circumstances can the treatment be labelled ordinary if it is morally obligatory or extraordinary if it is morally optional. (Furthermore, even if it is morally optional there remains a decision to be made by the patient or his proxies whether to carry it out.)

Burdensomeness of treatment

Of course, the criteria for assessing whether a proposed treatment is disproportionately burdensome are not precise, especially as laid down in the papal statement, which requires that the proposed life preserving treatments, in the "circumstances of persons, places, times, and cultures ... do not involve any great burden for oneself or another." One American authority on Roman Catholic medical ethics has interpreted this to mean that extraordinary means are those that cannot be obtained or used without excessive expense, pain, or other inconvenience or that do not offer a reasonable hope of success.[11] The Sacred Congregation's Declaration on Euthanasia says that in assessing burdensomeness the type of treatment, its risk and cost, and the difficulties of using it should be compared with the result to be expected, "taking into account the state of the sick person and his or her physical and moral resources." Patients may justifiably reject "a technique which is already in use but which carries a risk or is burdensome" and such rejection should be considered not as the equivalent of suicide but as an acceptance of the human condition, a wish to avoid the application of a medical procedure disproportionate to the expected results, or a desire not to impose excessive expense on the family or community.[4]

Burdens on others may be relevant

Understood thus the doctrine would surely be uncontroversial to most practising doctors, regardless of their religious faith or lack of it. Part of its uncontroversialness, however, lies precisely in its vagueness. What is meant by "disproportionately" or "excessively" burdensome? Whose opinion is to count when there is disagreement? Are some means always proportionate and thus morally obligatory or ordinary? In particular, is feeding always morally obligatory? When does the distinction apply? This is not the place to go into the considerable debate within the Roman Catholic church over these issues: suffice it to note that there seems to be general agreement that the patient's interests and perception of those interests are the primary moral consideration but that he and his proxies are morally permitted, perhaps even morally obliged, to take account not only of the burdens a proposed treatment would place on himself but also of the burdens it would impose on others.

There seems to be disagreement, however, about whether certain treatments are always morally obligatory, and especially so when the treatment is simply nourishment. Yet if the principle is accepted that the moral assessment must always be made in relation to the particular circumstances of a particular patient then it should always be possible in principle for a given means of treatment not to be morally obligatory, however common its use. This principle is widely accepted by Roman Catholic commentators in relation to such simple and widely available treatments as antibiotics (which may, it is widely agreed, be properly withheld from, for example, people who are already dying or who will soon die—the "old man's friend" approach[12]). Yet the logic of the underlying position seems to be too much for some commentators to stomach when it comes to the possibility of considering feeding as extraordinary or morally optional in particular cases. Thus Father John Mahoney SJ seems to reject the possibility that nourishment may be properly discontinued in any circumstances. Arguing that if ordinary feeding is impossible or extremely uncomfortable it may be discontinued "and attention switched to other possible means of nourishment," he goes on: "But nourishment itself, it appears, cannot be classed as medical 'treatment' to be assumed or discontinued, if only because to deprive a person of nourishment is more of the nature of undermining his resources and actively contributing to his death than of simply permitting his illness to take its course."[13]

May nutrition be withheld?

This view is widespread but not universal within the Roman

Catholic church. Thus Father John Parris SJ, writing in collaboration with a professor of paediatrics and criticising the then proposed American "Baby Doe" regulations requiring that nutrition and fluids be provided to every infant no matter how incurably and severely defective or diseased, argued that there are certain limited circumstances "in which nourishment and fluids may be entirely futile treatment."[14] Anencephaly and severe brain damage were offered as examples of such futility. Total necrotising enterocolitis was also offered as an example in which intravenous feeding would be inappropriate, despite the likely considerable prolongation of such an infant's life. The reasoning here, it seems clear from the context, is that because the infant would be committed to intravenous feeding for the rest of its life (at least until such time as bowel transplants became a clinical reality) such a treatment would be excessively burdensome.

The doctrine of ordinary and extraordinary means is misleadingly named, and some Roman Catholics prefer to speak of "proportionate" and "disproportionate" means.[4] When stripped of its misleading nomenclature, however, it provides reasonable non-absolutist guidance on how much doctors should strive to keep their patients alive. Essentially the answer is based on respect for the patient's own assessment of whether the struggle to stay alive would entail acceptable or excessive burdens, taking into account not just burdens on himself but those on his family and others. When such assessment is unavailable then his legitimate proxies should make the same assessment on his behalf. Such an approach is entirely consistent with a secular moral pluralist's assessment based on the principles of respect for autonomy, beneficence, non-maleficence, and justice. Nor does it seem to be radically different from the sorts of assessment of harm and benefit advocated by sophisticated utilitarians or from the assessments of harm and benefit that lead some clinicians to advocate allowing severely handicapped infants to die when their parents and doctors reasonably believe that treatment is futile or excessively burdensome,[15] and even to advocate withholding of nutrition when its provision is reasonably believed to be either futile or excessively burdensome.[16 17]

The final assessment

Of course, in particular cases there may be vigorous divergence of opinion about the final assessment. Roman Catholic opinion is, for example, widely, perhaps universally, opposed to the sort of letting die in which rejected infants with Down's syndrome are not fed and sedated and not given straightforward, life saving operations such as relief of duodenal atresia.[6 7 10 14 18 19] My impression, however, is that when there is a difference between thoughtful Roman Catholic and thoughtful non-Catholic thinking in such cases it often results from different weightings of the harms and benefits concerned in specific cases rather than from fundamental disagreement about the appropriate moral approach to such decision making—an approach which it is widely agreed requires that medical attempts to preserve people's lives should be regarded as an extremely important good, which it is morally important to pursue except when to do so is either futile or causes disproportionate harm.

References

1 President's Commission for the Study of Ethical Problems in Medicine. *Deciding to forgo life sustaining treatment*. Washington: US Government Printing Office, 1983:82-90.
2 Working Party of Linacre Centre. *Euthanasia and clinical practice—trends, principles and alternatives*. London: Linacre Centre, 1984:40-2. (Report.)
3 Pope Pius XII. The prolongation of life. In: Reiser SJ, Dyck AJ, Curran WJ, eds. *Ethics in medicine—historical perspectives and contemporary concerns*. Cambridge, Massachusetts; London: MIT Press, 1977:501-4.
4 Sacred Congregation for the Doctrine of the Faith. Declaration on euthanasia. In: *Deciding to forgo life sustaining treatment*. Washington: US Government Printing Office, 1983:300-7.
5 This claim, like most philosophical claims, is debated. A useful introductory collection of arguments, including the editor's introduction, is In: Hudson WD, ed. *The is/ought question*. London: Macmillan, 1969.
6 Linacre Centre. *Prolongation of life. 3. Ordinary and extraordinary means of prolonging life*. London: Linacre Centre, 1979.
7 Working Party of Linacre Centre. *Euthanasia and clinical practice—trends, principles and alternatives*. London: Linacre Centre, 1984:37-49. (Report.)
8 Dunstan GR. Life, prolongation of: ordinary and extraordinary means. In: Duncan AS, Dunstan GR, Welborn RB, eds. *Dictionary of medical ethics*. London: Darton Longman and Todd, 1981:266-8.
9 Reich WT, Ost DE. Ethical perspectives on the care of infants. In: Reich WT, ed. *Encyclopedia of bioethics*. London and New York: Collier Macmillan, 1978:724-42.
10 Mahoney J. *Bioethics and belief*. London: Sheed and Ward, 1984:36-51.
11 Kelly G. *Medico-moral problems*. St Louis: Catholic Hospital Association of the United States and Canada, 1958:128-41.
12 Mahoney J. *Bioethics and belief*. London: Sheed and Ward, 1984:45.
13 Mahoney J. *Bioethics and belief*. London: Sheed and Ward, 1984:46.
14 Paris JJ, Fletcher AB. Infant Doe regulations and the absolute requirement to use nourishment and fluids for the dying infant. *Law, Medicine and Health Care* 1983;11:210-3.
15 Campbell AGM. The right to be allowed to die. *J Med Ethics* 1983;9:136-40.
16 Campbell AGM. Children in a persistent vegetative state. *Br Med J* 1984;289:1022-3.
17 Lynn J, Childress JF. Must patients always be given food and water? *Hastings Center Report* 1983;5:17-21.
18 McCormick RA. To save or let die—the dilemma of modern medicine. *JAMA* 1974;229:172-6.

19 Paris JJ, McCormick RA. Saving defective infants: options for life or death. *America* 1983;**148**: 313-7.

Bibliography

Paris JJ, Reardon FE. Court responses to withholding or withdrawing artificial nutrition and fluids. *JAMA* 1985;**253**(15):2243-5. (A useful summary of American legal approaches to this problem.)

CHAPTER 23

On sickness and on health

Part of the moral defence of Dr Arthur was based on the differentiation of various functions of the doctor: to preserve the lives of his or her patients, to restore or preserve their health, and relieve, prevent, or minimise their pain and suffering. In this chapter I shall consider briefly what we mean by health and the relation of health to what is usually considered its contrary—namely, ill health, especially those varieties of ill health we call illness and disease. I shall focus on aspects of these broad philosophical issues that seem particularly important in medical ethics.

Perhaps the best known definition of health is that of the World Health Organisation (WHO), according to which "health is a state of complete physical, mental, and social wellbeing and not merely the absence of disease or infirmity."[1] According to this definition, none of us is, has ever been, or is ever likely to be healthy. Thus it does not leave much scope for doctors to restore or preserve the health of their patients, as none of them will ever have had it to restore or preserve. If, however, we modify the requirement of the WHO definition so that the doctor's function is to help to achieve the health of his patients then his function becomes extremely wide,[2] for it will be to try to help people to achieve "a state of complete physical, mental, and social wellbeing," and everyone who has not achieved that ideal state—that is, everyone—becomes not healthy and a potential patient. Imagine all the causes of one's incomplete physical mental or social wellbeing—including lack of preseason physical training, inadequate understanding of arithmetic or astrophysics, not enough money, social status, or lovers—becoming the legitimate concern of doctors.

Inadequacy of WHO definition of health

Either the stated function of doctors or the broad definition of health requires modification, and there seem to be good grounds for modifying both. Firstly, the definition of health. Despite the etymology of the word "healthy," which derives from the Old English for "whole" (as does the cognate "hale"), we simply do not mean we are in a state of complete wellbeing when we say we are healthy. Rather we mean that we are in a state of adequate or sufficient wellbeing. The state of complete wellbeing described in the WHO account may be an ideal at which to aim, but it is not a definition of health if we accept that there are, in fact, plenty of healthy people about enjoying a state of wellbeing of which unhealthy people are deprived.

Even if we accept some modification of the WHO definition such that health is a state of *adequate* physical, mental, and social wellbeing, the definition still seems too broad for any account of medicine's functions which includes preservation or restoration of health, let alone achievement of health. This is because people achieve, maintain, and restore an adequate physical mental and social wellbeing—that is, health according to this modified definition —by various means, as I have indicated above. If to call something medical is to indicate that it is the appropriate concern of doctors then only some of those means would plausibly be regarded as medical. How are we to distinguish within the broad concept of health that aspect or subsector of health or wellbeing that is the appropriate concern of doctors and other health care professionals? One strategy might be to argue that any aspects of health with which doctors *et al* do as a matter of fact concern themselves are properly called medical aspects of health. This implies that any concern of doctors is properly called medical and is likely to be rejected by those outside the profession as "medical imperialism"—the "expropriation of health" as Illich puts it[3]—and by those inside the profession as simply false.

Another approach is to differentiate the medical sphere of health concerns by reference to the sorts of impairments of health that are caused by ill health, notably illness and disease. On this account doctors would have the duty to restore and preserve those aspects of adequate wellbeing that have been impaired or are threatened by illness and disease. This seems to be getting closer to delineating the sorts of health concerns with which doctors are typically concerned and might avoid the awesome extension of a doctor's legitimate concerns into every aspect of human flourishing.

Realist and nominalist approaches

The problem then shifts to what we mean by ill health and its component concepts such as illness and disease. Such questions are extensively discussed (see bibliography), but two issues of particular relevance to medical ethics are the debate between realists and nominalists over whether there are such "things" as diseases, and the debate between those who argue that disease is necessarily an evaluative concept and those who claim that disease is a scientific concept free of values.

The first debate, at least in name, alludes to a hardy perennial of philosophical inquiry concerning the nature of universals—those properties of things that they share with other similar things.[4] If we accept the idiosyncratic use of realist/nominalist terminology in the debate about disease realists believe that the universal term "disease" refers to different types of entity or agent that cause different illnesses. Nominalists, on the other hand, such as Scadding and his colleagues, do not believe that there are such things as diseases, but that in medical discourse the name of a disease refers to "the sum of the abnormal phenomena displayed by a group of living organisms in association with a specified common characteristic or set of characteristics by which they differ from the norm of their species in such a way as to place them at a biological disadvantage."[5]

Apart from its intrinsic interest and the need for doctors to agree about what they mean when they use the term disease,[6] this debate is of some importance to medical ethics. One reason is that there exists, as Kennedy has noted, a tendency (though by no means a requirement) for realists to concentrate excessively on diseases and to fail to consider the whole person having the disease in his or her particular social context and environment.[7] On the other hand, nominalists risk the sort of subjectivism to which I have already referred—disease is simply whatever doctors decide is disease—indeed extreme nominalism leads to the extreme subjectivism of Humpty Dumpty: "Words mean what I chose them to mean."[4] Thus for the nominalist the potential scope of the concept of disease is exceedingly broad and can encompass a wide variety of what most would regard as non-medical "abnormal phenomena," which place people at "a biological disadvantage." For instance, as Toon points out,[8] under the above definition celibacy would count as a disease and, as Scadding *et al* cheerfully admit, so would poverty. Indeed it seems to me that even outstanding courage—for example, in battle—would count as a disease for is it not an abnormal phenomenon associated with specified common characteristics whereby its possessors differ from the norm of their species in such a way as to place them at a biological disadvantage? Scadding *et al* seek to overcome such objections to their definition by adding the discriminator (not in their definition but in their paper) of whether or not it is "useful" to define constellations of abnormal phenomena as diseases.[5] In what sense useful, useful to whom, and according to whom, we must ask?

Evaluation of disease

Such questions make clear how closely related the first debate between realism and nominalism is to the second one between those who regard disease as a value free concept and those who see it as necessarily evaluative. Scadding and his colleagues seem to be logically committed to a necessarily evaluative concept of disease. Thus the concept of "biological disadvantage" in their definition is evaluative, as is the concept of "useful," which they advocate as a discriminator for determining when constellations of abnormal phenomena that could be regarded as diseases should be so regarded.

A few stalwarts do argue that the concept of disease is value free (differentiating it from, for example, the concept of illness, in which the person's own evaluation of his symptoms plays an essential part). Thus Boorse argues that the concepts of both health and disease are non-evaluative and to be defined in terms of typical functioning for any particular species.[9] Health is analogous to the "perfect mechanical condition" of a motor car when it "conforms in all respects to the designer's detailed specifications": disease is "deviation from the natural functional organisation of the species" and a natural function is "nothing but a standard causal contribution to a goal actually pursued by the organism." I cannot do justice to his arguments here. Suffice it to say that they seem to entail either that any atypical functioning is a disease (the high jumper who clears 6 feet would then be diseased) or else that value laden concepts must be smuggled in to restrict the range of atypical functioning that can be called disease—for example, Boorse refers to "deficiencies" in the functional efficiency of the body and to "the action of a hostile environment" to pick out certain sorts of atypical functioning that he regards as diseases.

Definition of malady

But we still have not arrived at a plausible account of disease if all we are prepared to say is that it includes abnormal phenomena and characteristics that are negatively evaluated. Poverty in a society may fit these criteria and yet most people would be reluctant to classify it as a disease or illness. Several additional criteria have been proposed in excellent chapters on maladies and mental maladies by the psychiatric/philosophical team of Culver and Gert.[10] The first is that the evil or harm suffered by a person who has a malady (the authors' generic term for disease, illness, disability, infirmity, and so on) must be caused by something that is integral to and not separate from the person affected. Here they invoke the concept of a distinct sustaining cause whereby a "person has a malady if and only if the evil he is suffering does not have a sustaining cause which is clearly distinct from the person."

On this account poverty is not a disease, being caused by a distinct sustaining cause (lack of money), removal of which would rapidly ameliorate the evils or harms suffered by the poor person. On the other hand, poverty can itself cause various conditions—for example, nutritional deficiency or reactive depression—that are integral to the person, do cause harms, are not sustained by a distinct sustaining cause, and are thus maladies. A second criterion of malady is that the evil or harm may be risked rather than actually suffered, thus accounting for hidden or "lanthanic" disease[11] such as symptomless cancer discovered, say, on routine chest radiography, or symptomless high blood pressure. A third criterion is that if the harm or risk of harm is caused by the person's own rational beliefs or desires, or both, it is not a malady—refusal of blood by a Jehovah's

Witness, participation in hang gliding, or outstanding courage in battle are thus not maladies even though they increase a person's risk of harm.

Culver and Gert do not pretend that their account of maladies is unproblematical, but they claim, and the claim seems justified, that it avoids many of the implausibilities and obscurities of earlier accounts. Moreover, it affords a unified account for physical and mental maladies. It is an account that repays thorough study. One important ambiguity that does seem to remain, however, is the question of whose evaluation is to count: the patient's, society's, or some combination. Even if one accepts the claim by Culver and Gert that the harms or evils suffered or risked by those who have maladies would be avoided by every rational person unless the person has good reason not to avoid them there is an obvious grey area where the person concerned may not consider the state a harm or evil and not wish to avoid it, while his or her society may disagree (some cases of narcotic addiction may provide an example[12][13]).

Question answered?

I have been unable even to outline an adequate answer to my question: What aspect of health is properly the concern of medicine and, more broadly, of the health care professions? I have, however, indicated what seem to be some important components of such an answer as well as at least one remaining grey area: Whose evaluation is to count, that of the person who has the disease or other malady, that of the doctor, or that of society?

Let me end by suggesting that as both the definition and ascription of illness and disease or malady are of such profound social importance and can literally make people's decisions invalid—for example, under the Mental Health Act—and can excuse them from working or, more generally, from keeping their contractual obligations and can even protect them from being punished for serious offences under the law, and as these decisions are necessarily evaluative, such decision making ought to be a cooperative venture between doctors and society: neither can legitimately make these decisions independently. Such cooperation is already manifested to some degree in certain legal and parliamentary processes but these are sporadic and tend to be resented by the medical profession. If the above claims are valid such resentment is

inappropriate, and mechanisms for better and more consistent
cooperation need to be developed both to bring the various health
care professions together to think about these questions and to bring
them and appropriate representatives of the societies of which they
are a part together for the same purpose.

References

1 World Health Organisation. Basic documents: preamble to the constitution of the World Health
   Organisation. In: Reiser SJ, Dyck AJ, Curran JC, eds. *Ethics in medicine*. Cambridge,
   Massachusetts and London: MIT Press, 1977:552.
2 Callahan D. The WHO definition of health. In: Mappes TA, Zembaty JS, eds. *Biomedical ethics*.
   New York: McGraw-Hill, 1981:203-11. (Hastings Center Studies 1973;1 (3):77-87.)
3 Illich I. *Limits to medicine. Medical nemesis: the expropriation of health*. London: Marion Boyars,
   1976.
4 Woozley AD. Universals. In: Edwards P, ed. *The encyclopedia of philosophy*. London and New
   York: Collier Macmillan, 1967:194-206.
5 Campbell EJM, Scadding JG, Roberts RS. The concept of disease. *Br Med J* 1979;ii:757-62.
6 Anonymous. The concept of disease [Editorial]. *Br Med J* 1979;ii:751-2.
7 Kennedy I. *The unmasking of medicine*. London: George Allen and Unwin, 1981:20-5.
8 Toon PD. Defining "disease"—classification must be distinguished from evaluation. *J Med Ethics*
   1981;7:197-201.
9 Boorse C. On the distinction between disease and illness. *Philosophy and Public Affairs* 1975;5
   (1):49-68.
10 Culver CM, Gert B. *Philosophy in medicine*. New York and Oxford: Oxford University Press,
   1982:64-125.
11 Feinstein AR. *Clinical judgment*. Baltimore: Williams and Wilkins, 1967:145-8.
12 ten Have H, Sporken P. Heroin addiction, ethics and philosophy of medicine. *J Med Ethics*
   1985;11:173-7.
13 Anonymous. Heroin, health and disease [Editorial]. *J Med Ethics* 1985;11:171-2.

Bibliography

Sigerist HE. *A history of medicine. I: Primitive and archaic medicine*. New York: Oxford University
   Press, 1967:125-80, 331-5, 441-64.
Engelhardt HT, Spicker SF, eds. *Evaluation and explanation in the biomedical sciences*. Dordrecht and
   Boston: Reidel, 1975. (Especially Toulmin S. Concepts of function and mechanism in medicine
   and medical science, and Engelhardt HT. The concepts of health and disease, with commentary
   by Kopelman L.)
Engelhardt HT, Spicker SF, eds. *Health, disease and causal explanations in medicine*. Dordrecht and
   Boston: Reidel, 1984.
Beauchamp TL, Walters L, eds. *Contemporary issues in bioethics*. Encino and Belmont, California:
   Dickenson, 1978. (Especially Kass LR. Regarding the end of medicine and the pursuit of health:
   99-108, Engelhardt HT. The disease of masturbation: values and the concept of disease: 109-13,
   and Sedgwick P. What is illness? 114-9.)
Journal of Medicine and Philosophy 1976;1:201-80. (Monothematic issue on health and disease,
   especially Margolis J. The concept of disease: 238-55 and Redlich FC. Editorial reflections on the
   concepts of health and disease: 269-80.)
Journal of Medicine and Philosophy 1984;9:231-59. (Especially Hawkins A. Two pathographies: a
   study in illness and literature: 231-52, with commentary by Hudson-Jones A: 257-9, and Shelp
   EE. The experience of illness: integrating metaphors and the transcendence of illness: 253-6.)

Sontag S. *Illness as metaphor*. Harmondsworth: Penguin, 1977.

Dubos R. *Mirage of health*. London: George Allen and Unwin, 1960.

Mitchell J. *What is to be done about illness and health? Crisis in the eighties*. Harmondsworth: Penguin, 1984.

Engelhardt HT, Spicker SF, eds. *Mental health: philosophical perspectives*. Dordrecht and Boston: Reidel, 1978.

Edwards RB, ed. *Psychiatry and ethics*. Buffalo: Prometheus Books, 1982. (Various relevant papers on the concepts of mental health and disease, especially Szacz TS. The myth of mental illness: 19-28, Edwards RB. Mental health as rational autonomy: 68-78, and Engelhardt HT. Psychotherapy as metaethics: 61-7.)

Foucault M. *Madness and civilisation—a history of insanity in the age of reason*. London: Tavistock Publications, 1967.

Szacz T. *Ideology and insanity*. London: Penguin, 1974.

Journal of Medicine and Philosophy 1977;2:191-304. (Monothematic issue on mental health.)

Journal of Medicine and Philosophy 1980;5. (Monothematic issue on social and cultural perspectives on disease, especially Young A. An anthropological perspective on medical knowledge, and Unschuld PU. Concepts of illness in ancient China: the case of demonological medicine.)

Hastings Center Studies 1973;1(3). (Issue on the concept of health).

Journal of Medicine and Philosophy 1985;4:(several articles on diseases and maladies).

Hare RM. Health. *Journal of medical ethics* 1986;12(iv):(in press).

CHAPTER 24

"The patient's interests always come first?" Doctors and society

That doctors have a special moral obligation to their patients has been a recurrent theme in this series, and one to which I shall return in the next chapter. In this chapter I wish to pursue briefly some implications for medical ethics of the social context in which doctors practise. Such implications often contradict a common and absolutist medicomoral cliché that "the patient's interests always come first."

In earlier chapters I have indicated how even if doctors are interested only in the welfare of their own patients there may be times when moral obligations to others supersede their moral obligations to a particular patient. The most obvious example is when a doctor can satisfy one patient's requirements only at the expense of another's. Such examples multiply when the interests of one doctor's, specialty's, hospital's, or health authority's patients are incompatible with the interests of some other group of patients, and some principle of justice is needed to decide which patients' interests are to come first, and which are not. Given the vigorous disagreement among doctors and within our society generally about how to resolve such conflicts, given that doctors have no special skill in the matter, and given that most of the resources for satisfying the interests of any patients are being provided by a democratic society, there seems little doubt that society's representatives should be closely concerned with making these decisions, and indeed the structures for such decision making increasingly ensure this.

Similar considerations apply when we look at the potential medicomoral gap between the medical profession's obligations to its (collective) patients and the interests of sick people in general. The profession has long asserted in its official ethical codes that a doctor's primary moral obligation is to his patients,[1 2] and although it avows a principle of "service to humanity"[2 3] and even that "it is the mission of the medical doctor to safeguard the health of the people,"[4] it is clear that "the health of my patient will be my first consideration."[2] Although such medicomoral priority for our patients is laudable, it tends to leave people who are not patients out in the cold, often literally, and societies have become increasingly concerned to develop systems to ensure that all sick people can become patients and thus obtain the special moral concern of the medical profession. Nevertheless, vast areas of the world remain virtually without doctors, and in others, including our own, the distribution of medical services is uneven and the medical care of "the people" suffers accordingly.[5] Even if it is unrealistic to expect the medical profession to take seriously the sort of transnational moral obligation to all sick people extolled by Sir Theodore Fox in his Harveian oration[6] (which would certainly demand a radical restructuring of our attitudes, including perhaps some sort of compulsory international medical service during professional training to meet such an obligation to the otherwise undoctored sick) we should at least acknowledge sympathetically a legitimate area of social concern to achieve equitable distribution of medical care.

Society versus obligations to patients

In practice the medical profession accepts, at least implicitly, a broad range of social obligations that may override the interests of individual patients. The British Medical Association groups doctors' professional relationships into three categories[7]: therapeutic, impartial expert, and (non-therapeutic) medical researcher. The category of the medical researcher is implicitly justified by allowing medical obligations to non-existent patients of the future to take priority over medical obligations to existing patients. Preventative medicine (regarded by the BMA as an aspect of "impartial expert" medical work) implicitly acknowledges that medical concern for potentially sick people may in some circumstances take priority over therapeutic medicine. If the profession really believed that the patient's interests always come first then it presumably would not allow medical time and effort to be diverted away from direct therapeutic activity.

Quite apart from acknowledging that obligations to other patients, sick people, sick people in the future, and even merely potentially sick people may conflict with obligations to current patients, the medical profession also acknowledges implicitly that other legitimate demands of society may sometimes override doctors' obligations to their patients. In my discussion of medical confidentiality I outlined several exceptions, including legal requirements, in which, according to the British Medical Association and the General Medical Council, the patient's interest could legitimately be subordinated to the interests of society. When doctors ration scarce lifesaving medical resources (such as renal dialysis) they subordinate the patient's interests to those of society. When mentally sick patients are locked up against their will under the Mental Health Act because they are a danger to others the patient's interests are subordinated to those of society. Other examples include a wide range of medical interventions designed to protect society, such as medical examinations for driving and flying licences, military medical assessment of fitness to fight,[8] and medical examination of police suspects to detect drunkenness and excess blood alcohol or illegal drugs and weapons hidden in various body orifices.

Thus the medical profession does at least implicitly accept in practice that though its members have a strong obligation to their patients this is not an absolute obligation and may in some circumstances be overridden by their obligations to society. But despite this acceptance doctors often talk and think as if they believe that they invariably give absolute moral priority to their patients over the moral demands of society, as if indeed "the patient's interests always come first." It is a contradiction that needs to be confronted openly.

There certainly is a case to be made for doctors to give an absolute moral priority to their individual patients, but it carries with it various implications. Among these are the rejection of the currently accepted medical practices indicated above in which doctors do in fact give moral priority to their social obligations and acceptance that when conflict between the requirements of patients and those of others does arise non-medical individuals or organisations should be given the task of weighing up the competing claims fairly to try to ensure that justice is done.

Alternatively, the profession may decide to acknowledge that it does have moral obligations to the various social networks of which it is a part and that it is obliged to balance these obligations against its obligations to its individual patients and its members. Such weighing up is not easy, but a necessary condition for doing it is that the profession makes itself aware of what the various competing moral demands made by society on it actually are. That too is a difficult task, given that there is no single entity "society" but only a complex interlinking network of relationships between groups of people. It would surely be made easier if the profession welcomed, far more than it already does, into its deliberations about its moral obligations various representatives of these networks, as well as those whose professional expertise includes understanding these social networks and their interaction.

Medicine's hidden relations with society

Three more hidden aspects of medicine's relation with society are worth special mention as being at least indirectly relevant to medical ethics—and possibly leading to conflict with the interests of the individual patient. The first is the contribution of social factors to the causation of disease and illness, health, and wellbeing. The second is the contribution of social factors to doctors' attitudes about a wide range of issues, not least to their attitudes about medical ethics. The third is the struggle for power between the medical profession and other social groups.

The first of these aspects is relevant to medical ethics as it indicates an area of appropriate medicomoral concern that is widely ignored by the medical profession. If death, disease, and illness are caused by social factors; if changes in these social factors are both possible and can prevent or ameliorate these maladies; and if doctors as a profession are morally committed to these objectives then it follows that part of the medical profession's moral obligation is to understand and try to prevent the social causes of death, disease, and ill health.[9 11] It is, of course, an obligation that is well appreciated by some sectors of the profession, as shown by medical concern with, for example, the medical effects of nuclear warfare,[12-17] poverty and social class,[5 18 19] unemployment,[20 21] etc.

The second sociological factor of relevance to medical ethics is the influence of class on the medical profession's collective and individual attitudes. For example, even decisions about what abnormalities are classified as diseases are in part determined by social evaluations and it seems clear that doctors' evaluations are likely to fall within the norms of the ruling class, whatever it happens to be. Recall Professor Engelhardt's charming example of "drapetomania": a "disease" spotted by a doctor in the American south which caused slaves to keep running away from their masters.[22] In a plural society it seems particularly important to be aware of such socially determined attitudes, which are usually hidden, and to heed the warnings provided by such obviously unacceptable medical assumption of ruling class norms as in Nazi Germany,[23] Chile,[24] South Africa,[25] and Russia.[26] Nor need such hidden sociological influences on medical attitudes be dramatic ones to be resented by those who do not share them—medical assumptions of class superiority were criticised in a Department of Health and Social Security report on the doctor patient relationship.[27] Although there is enormous variation among doctors, it is probably reasonable to say that in Britain medical norms are biased towards those of the white middle class conservative Englishman.

There is nothing necessarily wrong with such norms, but nor is there anything necessarily right with them. Like all other attitudinal norms, they need to be assessed critically. To do so the first requirement is to discover what they are, for in many cases we are simply unaware of them, or of their power. Only when we have become aware of them can we give them the critical assessment that we expect and wish to give to the overt social demands made on us as a profession—for example, by parliament, the law, the media, and pressure groups.

Finally, the fairly powerful sociological status of doctors and the medical profession is likely to have important effects on our behaviour and the behaviour of others towards us. We need to understand, for example, the self interested and power maintaining aspects of our professional norms and rigorously avoid conflating them with aspects aimed at protecting patients.[28][29] When, for example, we insist that doctors must not advertise their services both components are present,[30] and in relation to medical ethics professional self interest is of comparatively little weight. Sociological investigations, aggravating though they may be, are surely a necessary antidote to a professional tendency for complacency and self deception about what we as a profession are really doing, and perceived to be doing. The debate between those who, like George Bernard Shaw, see the profession as a conspiracy against society[31] and those who, like Robert Louis Stevenson, see doctors as the flower of all mankind[32] continues unabated.[33 40] As usual, there is some truth in both points of view; while many doctors doubtless prefer Stevenson's account, it is important to understand how and why our behaviour as a profession provokes such rejection as it does.

Social and psychological influences on medical ethics

I should perhaps end by addressing a likely objection. At the outset of this book I declared that philosophical medical ethics was not a sociological, psychological, anthropological, historical, or religious enterprise, yet here I appear to be leaning heavily on such perspectives. There is no contradiction. Although I stand by the original claim, in pursuing the "critical evaluation of assumptions and arguments" that is at the heart of philosophical inquiry it is important to be aware of the genesis of those assumptions, which so often form the premises of the arguments under assessment. We know, for example, that some social and cultural loyalties and pressures, some religious attitudes, and some psychological factors (including some aspects of self interest and partiality) can lead people to beliefs, assumptions, and arguments, moral and otherwise, which more detached analysis repudiates. To distinguish between the acceptable and the unacceptable variants of such social and psychological determinants it helps to be aware of both their existence and of their characteristics.

References

1 British Medical Association. *Handbook of medical ethics*. London: BMA, 1984:69.
2 British Medical Association. *Handbook of medical ethics*. London: BMA, 1984:70-2.
3 British Medical Association. *Handbook of medical ethics*. London: BMA, 1984:78-80.
4 British Medical Association. *Handbook of medical ethics*. London: BMA, 1984:43-6.
5 Black DAK, Morris JN, Smith C, Townsend P, Davidson N. *Inequalities in health: the Black report*. Harmondsworth: Penguin, 1982.
6 Fox T. Purposes of medicine. *Lancet* 1965;ii:801-5.
7 British Medical Association. *Handbook of medical ethics*. London: BMA, 1984:11.
8 Beauchamp TL, Childress JF. *Principles of biomedical ethics*. 2nd ed. Oxford and New York: Oxford University Press, 1983:242-3.
9 McKeown T. *The role of medicine: dream, mirage or nemesis?* London: Nuffield Provincial Hospitals Trust, 1976.

10 Illsley R. *Professional or public health?* London: Nuffield Provincial Hospitals Trust, 1980.
11 Fitzpatrick RM. Social causes of disease. In: Patrick DL, Scambler B, eds. *Sociology as applied to medicine.* London: Ballière Tindall, 1982:30-40.
12 Chivian E, ed. *Last aid: the medical dimensions of nuclear war.* Oxford: W H Freeman, 1982.
13 International physicians for the prevention of nuclear war. Call for an end to the nuclear arms race. *Lancet* 1983;ii:506.
14 British Medical Association. *Report of the Board of Science and Education inquiry into the medical effects of nuclear war.* London: BMA, 1983.
15 Relman AS. Physicians, nuclear war and politics. *N Engl J Med* 1982;**307**:744-5.
16 Haines A, White CB, Gleisner J. Nuclear weapons and medicine: some ethical dilemmas. *J Med Ethics* 1983;**9**:200-6.
17 Kay HEM. Thinking the unthinkable at Easingwold. *Lancet* 1984;i:38-9.
18 Mullan F. *White coat, clenched fist: the political education of an American physician.* New York: Macmillan, 1976.
19 Blane D. Inequality and social class. In: Patrick DL, Scambler B, eds. *Sociology as applied to medicine.* London: Baillière Tindall, 1982:113-24.
20 Smith R. Occupationless health. *Br Med J* 1985;**291**:1024-7, 1107-11, 1191-5, 1263-6, 1338-41, 1409-12, 1492-5, 1563-6, 1626-9, 1707-10.
21 Higgs R. Unemployment in my practice: Walworth, London. *Br Med J* 1981;**283**:532. (One of a series of articles on this theme by general practitioners, starting at 282:2020-1 and ending at 283:1844-5.)
22 Engelhardt HT. The concepts of health and disease. In: Engelhardt HT, Spicker SF, eds. *Evaluation and explanation in the biomedical sciences.* Dordrecht: Reidel, 1975:138.
23 Ivy AC. Nazi war crimes of a medical nature. Reprinted in: Reiser SJ, Dyck AJ, Curran WJ, eds. *Ethics in medicine—historical perspectives and contemporary concerns.* Cambridge, Massachusetts and London: MIT Press, 1977:267-72.
24 Jadresic A. Doctors and torture: an experience as a prisoner. *J Med Ethics* 1980;**6**:124-7.
25 Tobias PV. South African Medical and Dental Council and the "Biko doctors." *Br Med J* 1980;**251**:231.
26 Bloch S, Reddaway P. *Soviet psychiatric abuse: the shadow over world psychiatry.* London: Victor Gollancz, 1984.
27 Fitton F, Acheson HWK. *The doctor/patient relationship: a study in general practice.* London: HMSO, 1979.
28 Jefferys M. Independence and the GP: retrospect and prospect. *Update* 1985;**31**:733-6.
29 Berlant JL. *Profession and monopoly—a study of medicine in the United States and Great Britain.* Berkeley, Los Angeles, London: University of California Press, 1975.
30 Dyer AR. Ethics advertising and the definition of a profession. *J Med Ethics* 1985;**11**:72-8.
31 Shaw GB. *The doctor's dilemma.* London: Bodley Head, 1973.
32 Stevenson RL. Underwoods. In: Smith JA, ed. *Collected poems.* London: Rupert Hart-Davis, 1950.
33 Kennedy I. *The unmasking of medicine.* London: Allen and Unwin, 1981.
34 Anonymous. Medicine, profession and society [editorial]. *J Med Ethics* 1985;**11**:59-60.
35 Sieghart P. Professions as the conscience of society. *J Med Ethics* 1985;**11**:117-22.
36 Downie R. Professional ethics. *J Med Ethics* 1986;**12**:64-65.
37 Sieghart P. Professional ethics: reply to Professor Downie. *J Med Ethics* 1986;**12**:66.
38 Gillon R. More on professional ethics [editorial]. *J Med Ethics* 1986;**12**:59-60.
39 Downie R. Professional ethics: further comments. *J Med Ethics* 1986;**12**(iv) (in press).
40 Gillon R. Professional ethics: a response to Professor Downie. *J Med Ethics* 1986;**12**(iv) (in press).

CHAPTER 25

Doctors and patients

In the last chapter and intermittently throughout this book I have suggested that doctors do not have an overriding duty to benefit their patients, and that sometimes moral obligations to others will supersede this duty. That of course does not conflict with what to doctors is the obvious claim that they do have special, supererogatory, moral obligations to their patients—that is, moral obligations that are over and above the ordinary moral obligations we all have to each other.

In this chapter I shall outline some prima facie moral duties of doctors to their patients that emerge from my preceding discussions of philosophical medical ethics. Their importance seems to stem from the fact that they follow from four general ethical principles that various moral theories would accept, plus the special self imposed supererogatory duty of beneficence that doctors as members of the medical profession profess. I have tried in preceding chapters to point to the complexity and some of the nuances underlying these principles. Here I shall try to summarise their prima facie implications more baldly and boldly with less philosophical circumspection, but I shall not discuss the manifold problems that arise when these obligations conflict. I suspect, however, that even the prima facie obligations will be startling and contentious enough for many doctors, though for others they may be self evident.

Respect for autonomy

Firstly, in their relationships with their patients doctors must remember that apart from any special moral obligations they have the standard moral obligations that all of us have to each other: to respect each other's autonomy, not to harm each other (non-maleficence), to be just, and to benefit at least some others (beneficence). The extent and nature of these last two general moral obligations are more debated than the first two, but in the absence of justification to the contrary they ought to be followed at least to the extent determined by our social, including legal, obligations.

In addition, doctors voluntarily take on an additional moral obligation—what might be called the principle of medical beneficence—to benefit their patients' health and to some extent the health of others. They undertake to do so by trying to save their patients' lives when these are threatened by disease and other "maladies" (in the sense used by Culver and Gert[1]); to cure, palliate, and prevent their maladies; and to ameliorate the suffering that these cause. If we accept our general moral obligations these additional duties of medical beneficence ought only to be exercised to the extent that our patients want and allow us to exercise them. Thus our general duty to respect their autonomy requires that if they do not want to be helped we generally have no right to help them (though I have previously outlined a rationale for certain exceptions to this norm). Even our general duty not to harm others requires for the most part that we try our best to obtain their willing consent to what we propose as most interventions designed to help others carry a risk of harming them and that risk is probably increased considerably if they are carried out without people's understanding and consent, let alone if they are carried out against their will.

If we add to these general moral obligations the special obligation of medical beneficence then our duty to respect our patients' autonomy should generally be reinforced; in most cases doctors will benefit their patients more if the rationale of their proposed beneficial actions is understood and approved by their patients. Respect for a patient's autonomy should thus be seen as a presupposition of the doctor-patient relationship, not only because it is the underlying assumption behind any voluntary interpersonal relationship but also because in any case such respect will probably improve the beneficent outcome that the doctor intends to produce.

Doctor-patient relationship

None the less, it is uncontroversial to assert that the principle of respect for autonomy has had little milage for most of medicine's long history except, perhaps, when patients have been doctors' social equals or superiors (Plato alluded to this distinction when he differentiated between the doctor-slave patient relationship, in which the patient did what the doctor told him to do without discussion and that was the end of the matter, and the doctor-rich citizen relationship, in which explanation and discussion were the norm[2]). The medical sociologist Dr Ann Cartwright is not alone when she says she likes her doctor to treat her "as an equal,"[3] but this is by no means a medical norm.

The implications for the doctor-patient relationship of taking the principle of respect for autonomy seriously are legion. Among the more important are the following prima facie duties: to give the patient at least what he or she considers to be adequate information, and often more if the doctor knows that more information will probably be appreciated and relevant to good decision making; not to lie to or otherwise deceive the patient (unless he or she deliberately chooses such deception); and to allow the patient to have at least strategic control over which course of action to pursue—that is, the doctor may advise, but the patient is then given the opportunity to decide whether to accept that advice. If this principle is taken seriously, a patient's rejection of medical advice should not lead to a shrugging of the shoulders, a cooling of attitude, and "if you can't trust my advice, perhaps you'd better find another doctor." What should follow instead is a genuine attempt to understand the patient's reasons (or other motives) for rejecting the advice and a search for the next best option.

One of the keys to respect for autonomy is good communication, and thus respect for patients' autonomy requires doctors to acquire and maintain skill in communicating with them—not just in telling but also in understanding.[4-13] As Sir George Pickering said in his Nuffield lecture, although a few doctors are born communicators, most are not, but they can learn[14] (and when such teaching is set up we need to incorporate the patients' assessments of the appropriate standards for "good" doctor-patient communication).

If respect for autonomy requires that we cannot treat people without their understanding consent then still less can we use them for the benefit of others without such consent, whether in research or medical teaching, and their refusal of such consent should not detract from their ordinary medical care. Even a prima facie obligation to be punctual stems from the requirement to respect autonomy (assuming the obligation to keep one's promises derives from the requirement to respect autonomy) because to offer someone an appointment is a form of promising).

An infinite range of other specific prima facie obligations derive from the principle of respect for autonomy, including, perhaps, the provision of more information about doctors' interests, qualifications, attitudes, and moral stances to patients and potential patients as well as making it as easy as possible for patients to have a real choice of doctor. There is often an unwritten agreement, especially among general practitioners, not to accept patients who wish to change from neighbouring doctors with whom they are dissatisfied. Respect for autonomy would seem at first sight to require otherwise. The same applies to the General Medical Council's advice that "in the interests of the generality of patients a specialist should not usually accept a patient without reference from the patient's general practitioner."[15] For the General Medical Council to precede this remark with the assertion that "an individual patient is free to seek to consult any doctor" is, to say the least, disingenuous, though it is presumably supposed to reflect the World Medical Association's affirmation in the Declaration of Lisbon,[16] subscribed to by Britain, that "the patient has the right to choose his physician freely." (Dissatisfaction with professional restrictions on advertising and restrictions on patients' choice of doctor have reached the leader columns of *The Times*).[17]

In summary, the principle of respect for autonomy asks the doctor to have at the back of his mind the question, Would the patient, if he could consider it, wish me to do what I am doing or intend to do? If not, How can I justify doing it? Usually the best way to answer the first question is to ask the person concerned.

Non-maleficence and beneficence

The second and third principles—that is, non-maleficence and beneficence—almost always need to be considered together in the context of the doctor-patient relationship, for although non-maleficence can be considered independently of beneficence, any obligation to help others that may result in harm, including almost any medical intervention, has to be considered in the context of the coexisting obligation not to harm others. Countless important prima facie medical obligations stem from these two principles, of which I shall indicate a few.

Firstly, if a doctor professes to be able and willing to benefit his patients then he or she had better *be* able and willing to do so; and as he is under a general obligation not to harm others he had better do so with minimal harm (the real force of the traditional "primum non nocere" slogan). This has straightforward implications for medical education before and throughout professional life for as members of a profession we are obliged (by accepting these two principles) to ensure that we practise in ways that do actually benefit our patients with minimal harm. This entails continual research to discover what these ways are, educating ourselves to practise in these ways, and continually monitoring our performance to make sure that we practise and continue to practise accordingly. Thus continuing postgraduate medical education, including some form of audit, is a moral obligation, as distinct from an optional extra taken on by enthusiasts, the sort of obligation that "springs from a mutual respect and a desire to improve the lot of patients."[18] (As the Royal College of General Practitioners[19] and Dr John Lister,[20] among others, have pointed out, there are also other, prudential reasons for the profession to undertake more rigorous self assessment of the quality of its service.)

What about medical mishaps? It seems that doctors—and I include myself—have a tendency to close ranks in their own individual and group interests and against the interests of our patients to an extent that is incompatible with our professed adherence to a principle of benefiting our patients. We have had inculcated into us throughout our professional training and socialisation a sort of public school ethos that we do not "split" about a colleague even when we know that the colleague has made a damaging mistake or is frankly incompetent (let alone when we merely know that he is unpleasant to his patients). Such behaviour is incompatible with the principle of medical beneficence that doctors profess, and if we are to continue honestly to profess it we need a radical new orientation to eliminate this tendency.

During a tour of various establishments that teach ethics in the United States, I visited West Point Military Academy, which teaches ethics to its cadets (and also to officers at various later stages in their careers). Part of the undergraduate teaching is carried out by the cadets themselves and includes among other components promulgation and justification of an "honour code." When I first discovered that this required cadets to report each other's moral misdemeanours of lying, cheating, and theft I was repelled by the sort of disloyalty and threat to friendship that such a code required. Just as the military (sexistly) speak of "brother officers" so the International Code of Medical Ethics affirms that "my colleagues will be my brothers"[21]; surely brothers do not report each other's misdemeanours unless they are really awful. On reflection, however, I am not so sure. Should not our professed medical ethic of benefiting our patients require something similar to the cadets' honour code? Should we not educate ourselves from student days onwards that our primary loyalty should be to our patients and if that conflicts with our personal and professional friendships and group loyalties, even with our loyalties to our medical "brothers," the prima facie assumption should be that the patients' interests come first?

Of course, ideally no doctor would deceive, cheat, or defraud his patients, nor in any other way harm them unnecessarily, but we do not live in an ideal world. I do not think my own personal reluctance to "dish a colleague" is rare within our profession—according to Sir Douglas Black, such reluctance was one of the themes emerging from a Royal College of Physicians' symposium on medical accountability[22]—yet if we are to take our self imposed moral obligation to benefit our patients seriously such reluctance should become rare. The case against medical in-group loyalty superseding loyalty to patients was argued powerfully by a solicitor who helped to found the organisation Action for the Victims of Medical Accidents.[23]

Admit mistakes to patients

While on this theme, I read with interest the assertion of a past president of the Law Society that "of the three true professions, it would seem overall that the ethical standards which are required of the lawyer exceed those of any other profession." Part of this claim rested on an aspect of legal practice that was "unlike any other profession"—notably, that solicitors "are obliged by the rules of professional conduct to inform a client if they have acted negligently or improperly in the performance of their work. This is not incumbent on ... the surgeon or physician who tends you in ill health. ..."[24] Admittedly, a solicitor friend had never heard of this fine self imposed obligation, but is it not entirely admirable and one that we as a profession committed to benefiting our patients should take up? Interestingly, it seems that the law may be nudging us in that direction, at least so far as answering patients' questions truthfully and completely is concerned, not only concerning proposed treatments (as in the judgments of Lords Keith and Bridge in the Sidaway case[25]) but also, in a more recent Court of Appeal case, concerning treatments that have already been given.[26]

If we do decide to accept the implication of the principle of medical beneficence, that we should tell patients if we have made mistakes, it would also be reasonable for us to press for a national scheme of no fault compensation. We are bound to make mistakes from time to time, some of which are bound to harm our patients, and compensation should not depend on a legal requirement to show "negligence." Nor if we are concerned with the ethics of the matter should we allow our legal protection societies to stop us apologising to our patients; if we think we have made a mistake we almost certainly have, and we should out of common decency, let alone the principle of medical beneficence, say we are sorry. This requirement may in any case be of considerable benefit to the doctor as well as to the victim of his mistake, as Dr Hilfiker points out in a wise and humble paper.[27]

Finally, in this consideration of the implications of beneficence, should we not build into medical training and standards a requirement to be nice to our patients? Doubtless it is true, as is heard over and over again in response to this suggestion, that, firstly, all doctors are nice to some of their patients some of the time and, secondly, patients would prefer a medically competent but unpleasant doctor to a charming ignoramus. But is the first sufficient if we profess beneficence and as for the second would not a combination of the two be even better? Being pleasant, warm, concerned, and, where appropriate, compassionate on the one hand and being medically and scientifically competent on the other are not mutually exclusive attributes.[28] Quite apart from any moral obligation of beneficence Dr Mendel suggests that we are paid to be nice to patients[29] (he also suggests that the short appointment is one of the worst enemies of "proper doctoring" in this and other respects), and doctors writing about their own experiences as patients indicate the importance they attached to the friendliness of their treatment, or its absence.[30-34]

My personal impression, however, reinforced by what I hear from my patients and the medical stories of my friends, is that doctors, and taking their cue from them staff throughout the National Health Service, including receptionists, have a propensity for retreating into a sort of dismissively neutral frame of mind and face, especially when patients show the slightest sign of dissatisfaction. Such lack of friendliness, aloofness, and inadequate communication from staff experienced and observed during Member of Parliament Mr Patrick McNair-Wilson's stay in hospital were apparently among the causes that prompted him to introduce his government supported Hospital Complaints Procedure Bill.[35] [36] Does not medical beneficence require at least a consistently friendly and pleasant medical demeanour?

I am not suggesting that we ought, or even that we could, become real friends with each of our patients; indeed strictly speaking the principle of beneficence requires no emotional ties at all (as distinct from a principle of benevolence that would require good feelings, beneficence requires only good actions). Some affection, some interest, and some genuine concern is, however, as a matter of empirical fact likely to make it easier for a doctor to be beneficent to his patients in all these different ways, and while there is a positive danger to medical care if the emotions play too large a part, so there is if they are cut out altogether. My impression is that as members of a profession we have strayed too far towards impersonality and detachment and that we need actively to correct the balance and encourage and foster the sort of "moderated love" for our patients described so well by the Scottish theologian Dr Alastair Campbell.[37]

Justice

Justice too should have its impact on the doctor-patient relationship. I indicated in my earlier chapters on justice the lack of agreement about which substantive principle of justice should be adopted, but I also indicated that most theorists would accept Aristotle's formal principle according to which equals should be treated equally and unequals treated unequally in proportion to the relevant inequality, and that that formal principle alone had substantive implications for medical care. Doctors simply cannot evade the conclusion that there are various circumstances in which the interests of others may supersede the interests of their index patient of the moment. But perhaps we need to make it clearer to our patients that although we work hard to support their interests, we also have obligations to others that on rare occasions may override their interests (perhaps not so rarely if it is an inchoate principle of distributive justice that allows doctors to provide the incredibly short consultations that on the whole are the unwelcome lot of so many NHS patients).

Professional codes of medical ethics such as those promulgated by the General Medical Council and the British Medical Association already indicate the many competing moral concerns that may override a doctor's primary obligation to his patient of the moment. As individual doctors, however, I think we tend to imply, if not actually say, to our patients that their particular welfare and interests are always paramount, their secrets are in absolute trust, whatever they medically need they will get, etc. Perhaps we should make it clearer that although we consider ourselves individually and collectively to have a strong obligation to each of our patients, we do not and could not purport to have an absolute obligation to them.

Perhaps we should also give them some indication or summary of our personal professional ethics and our approach to various standard medicomoral dilemmas, as the barrister Paul Sieghart suggested in his Lucas lecture.[38] Of course, the chances of the present generation of doctors actually doing this are remote, but a modest start could be made if some standard exposition such as the BMA handbook of ethics were available in every surgery and hospital firm, to be consulted by patients who were interested. Enthusiasts representing various standard and alternative medico-moral stances might consider writing explanatory handbooks for patients. Gradually it would become the norm for doctors to discuss medicomoral issues with those patients who wished to know if they were morally "compatible" with their doctors and to negotiate particular issues. I do not believe that this, even if it were widely available, would take up a large proportion of our time as doctors, nor should it. But the offer and ability to discuss critically and knowledgably such issues with our patients would greatly enhance the quality of our overall medical practice.

All the above implications of the four "standard" moral principles are prima facie and each applies only if one of the others does not supersede it. None the less, even as prima facie obligations they present a formidable set of requirements, and I do not delude myself that we can always live up to these duties even if we accept them. I certainly cannot, try as I may.

One conflicting motivation that I have not considered is self interest. To some degree self interest is a moral obligation in so far as it is also required to some degree by at least three of the four principles. Respect for autonomy, non-maleficence, and justice are moral obligations that extend to all, including ourselves. Moreover, if we flourish ourselves we are better able among other things to carry out our obligations to others, including our obligations to benefit our patients. Whether we have a duty of beneficence to ourselves independently of such considerations is more doubtful. Utilitarians would generally argue that we do to the extent that such self beneficence maximises overall welfare. Whether this is accepted, at the very least self beneficence (or looking after number one) needs to be distinguished carefully from the other moral obligations influencing the doctor-patient relationship. Certainly the special moral obligation that we profess of beneficence to our patients would seem to imply that when an uncomplicated conflict arises between benefiting them medically and benefiting ourselves then prima facie their interests should take priority. If it does not entail at least this what is left of our claims of being a profession?

References

1 Culver CM, Gert B. *Philosophy in medicine: conceptual and ethical issues in medicine and psychiatry.* New York, Oxford: Oxford University Press, 1982:64-108.
2 Plato. *Laws.* 720.
3 Cartwright A. Equality of experts. *Br Med J* 1983;287:538.
4 Fletcher CM. *Communication in medicine.* London: Nuffield Provincial Hospitals Trust, 1973.
5 Pendleton D, Hasler J, eds. *Doctor-patient communication.* London: Academic Press, 1983.
6 Katz J. *The silent world of doctor and patient.* London: Collier Macmillan, 1984.
7 Fitton F, Acheson HWK. *The doctor-patient relationship: a study in general practice.* London: HMSO, 1979.
8 Freeling P, Harris CM. *The doctor-patient relationship.* 3rd ed. Edinburgh, London, Melbourne, New York: Churchill Livingstone, 1984.
9 Locker D. Communication in general practice. In: Patrick DL, Scambler G, eds. *Sociology as applied to medicine.* London: Baillière Tindall, 1982.
10 Royal College of General Practitioners. *What sort of doctor? Assessing quality of care in general practice.* London: Royal College of General Practitioners, 1985.
11 Byrne PS, Long BEL. *Doctors talking to patients.* London: HMSO, 1976.
12 Cartwright A, Anderson R. *General practice revisited.* London: Tavistock Publications, 1981.
13 Stinson GV, Webb B. *Going to see the doctor: the consultation process in general practice.* London: Routledge and Kegan Paul, 1975.
14 Pickering G. Medicine at the crossroads. *Proceedings of the Royal Society of Medicine* 1977;70: 16-20.
15 General Medical Council. *Professional conduct and discipline: fitness to practise.* London: General Medical Council, 1985:23.
16 World Medical Association. Declaration of Lisbon: the rights of the patient. Reprinted in: British Medical Association. *The handbook of medical ethics.* London: British Medical Association, 1984:72-3.
17 Anonymous. Incentives in the surgery [Editorial]. *The Times* 1985 November 9:9.

18 McIntyre N, Popper K. The critical attitude in medicine: the need for a new ethics. *Br Med J* 1983;**287**:1919-23.
19 Royal College of General Practitioners. *Quality in general practice*. London: Royal College of General Practitioners, 1985:13-5.
20 Lister J. The British medical scene since 1980. *N Engl J Med* 1983;**308**:532-5.
21 World Medical Association. Declaration of Geneva. Reprinted in: British Medical Association. *The handbook of medical ethics*. London: British Medical Association, 1984:70.
22 Black D. Medical accountability. *J R Coll Physicians Lond* 1985;**19**:203-4.
23 Simanowitz A. Standards, attitudes and accountability in the medical profession. *Lancet* 1985;ii:546-7.
24 Napley D. The ethics of the professions. *The Law Society's Gazette* 1985;**82**:818-25.
25 Anonymous. Sidaway v Bethlem Royal Hospital and the Maudsley Hospital Health Authority and others [Law Report]. *The Times* 1985 February 22:28.
26 Anonymous. Lee v South West Thames Regional Health Authority. Court of Appeal. *New Law Journal* 1985 May 3:438-9.
27 Hilfiker D. Facing our mistakes. *N Engl J Med* 1984;**310**:118-22.
28 Black D. *An anthology of false antitheses*. London: Nuffield Provincial Hospitals Trust, 1984: 17-30.
29 Mendel D. *Proper doctoring*. Berlin, Heidelberg, New York, Tokyo: Springer-Verlag, 1984.
30 Hall A. Personal view. *Br Med J* 1985;**291**:1274.
31 Rabin ED, Rabin PL, Rabin R. Compounding the ordeal of ALS-isolation from my fellow physicians. *N Engl J Med* 1982;**307**:506-9.
32 Frank SE. Lessons. *JAMA* 1984;**252**:2014.
33 Townend M. Personal view. *Br Med J* 1985;**290**:462.
34 Burnfield A. Doctor-patient dilemmas in multiple sclerosis. *J Med Ethics* 1984;i:21-6.
35 Deitch R. An MP's charter for hospital patients. *Lancet* 1984;ii:824.
36 Deitch R. A Bill on patients' complaints introduced by an MP who was a patient. *Lancet* 1985;i:708.
37 Campbell AV. *Moderated love*. London: SPCK, 1984.
38 Sieghart P. Professional ethics—for whose benefit? *J Med Ethics* 1982;**8**:25-32.

Bibliography

Gorovitz S. *Doctors' dilemmas: moral conflict and medical care*. New York: Macmillan, 1982.
Walton J, McLachlan G, eds. *Doctor to doctor: writing and talking about patients*. London: The Nuffield Provincial Hospitals Trust, 1984.
Waitzkin H. Doctor-patient communication: clinical implications of social scientific research. *JAMA* 1984;**252**:2441-6.
Feinstein RJ. The ethics of professional regulation. *N Engl J Med* 1985;**312**:801-4.
Relman AS. Professional regulation and the state medical boards. *JAMA* 1985;**312**:784-6.
Kennedy I. Rethinking medical ethics. *J R Coll Surg Edinb* 1982;**27**:1-8.
Anonymous. Medical student selection in the UK [Editorial]. *Lancet* 1984;ii:1190-1.
Anonymous. City practice revealed: territorial rights. *Update* 1984 October 1:583-6.
Russell W. Drug addicts unwelcome patients, MPs told. *Br Med J* 1985;**290**:573.
Cook S. Blacks meet race bias from GPs. *The Guardian* 1983 March 28.
Ormrod Sir R. A lawyer looks at medical ethics. *Med Leg J* 1978;**46**:18-32.

CHAPTER 26

Conclusion:
The Arthur case revisited

I started this book with two moral arguments that stemmed from a well known legal case. One argument rejected as wrong Dr Arthur's prescribing of dihydrocodeine and "nursing care only" for a rejected newborn infant with Down's syndrome and the other defended what he did as right. Seeking to show the complexity of reasoning that should underlie the conclusions "he was right" or "he was wrong," I extracted many moral claims and assumptions made in each argument. In the subsequent chapters I analysed many of these. What, if any light can such analyses shed on those opposing arguments about the Arthur case? The first point is that these issues are exceedingly complex. Next it should be clear that rational arguments for each side of this case can be mounted by sincere people anxious to come to right conclusions. Thus it is inappropriate to assume stupidity, ignorance, or ill intent in those who reach opposing conclusions to one's own in medicomoral arguments.

An approach to moral dilemmas

In medicomoral dilemmas I have suggested looking at the relevance of the four principles outlined by Beauchamp and

Childress[1] and acceptable within a variety of moral theories. (Of course other methods could be and have been devised.[2][3]) These principles are respect for autonomy, beneficence, non-maleficence, and justice. I have also indicated that the moral analysis may sometimes turn on issues of scope—what moral duties do we have to this particular entity or type of entity? Whatever moral duties we may have to experimental rats, for example, we do not have to respect their autonomy, because rats cannot have autonomy and so cannot fall within the scope of respect for autonomy. In the Arthur case it seems to me that the crucial first moral question is indeed a question of scope: Do the same moral obligations that we have to our other patients extend to newborn infants with Down's syndrome? If the answer is yes our moral analysis will travel down the same path as in any moral dilemma concerning our patients—we will have the same sort of moral obligations to that newborn baby as we have to any other temporarily or permanently non-autonomous patient. If, on the other hand, the answer is no we do not have the same moral obligations to that baby as we have to our patients in general—suppose, for example, we have obligations more stringent than we have to a fetus but less stringent than we have to a young child—then our analysis will follow a different path, more like that followed when we consider our moral obligations to fetuses.

Moral decisions imposed by the nature of things

It seems that the scope of our moral obligations may be determined in several ways. Sometimes it is determined by individual and morally optional decisions; thus we can create self imposed moral obligations to some people and not others—for example, I may take on a previously non-existent moral obligation by promising one or more people that I will do something. Sometimes the scope of a moral obligation is determined by the morally optional decisions of a group of people. Such are the special moral obligations taken on by doctors, nurses, and lifeboatmen (and possibly clergy?). Sometimes the scope of a moral obligation is determined by the laws or customs of a particular society. One society may require its members to help the sick and poor, another may leave this to individual charity. One society may require children to look after their aging or sick parents, another may regard this as morally optional. I assume that the special moral obligations that we owe our family, neighbours, community, tribe, group, and nation are of this variable and socially determined kind.

Sometimes, however, the scope of our moral obligations seems not to be optional. Instead these obligations derive from the nature of certain sorts of entity. I take it that there is something about the nature of other people (including our patients) that we recognise to impose on us certain sorts of moral obligations, to require from us a certain sort of moral respect. We recognise, moreover, that we have no moral option about acknowledging these obligations. I take it that there is something different about the nature of waxworks, statues, or even dead bodies that allows us not to have the same moral obligations to them that we would acknowledge to the people they resemble (and, in the case of the bodies, were). Similarly, there is a morally relevant difference between pheasants and peasants which allows us to shoot one but not the other. Conversely, if there is no such difference then we are morally obliged to eschew such discrimination and be ready to shoot both or neither.

Which properties of things are morally relevant?

Such questions are crucial to discussion of a wide variety of medicomoral issues, including contraception, postcoital contraception, research on embryos, abortion, severe brain damage, persistent vegetative state, brain stem death, and traditional cardiorespiratory death. Characteristics of things that have been plausibly argued to be criteria for moral categorisation include membership of particular species, notably the human species, possession of the capacity to experience pain (sentience), and possession of the capacities of being a person, whatever those might be, but perhaps including the capacity of self awareness as a necessary condition. "Viability," arbitrary dates of gestation, and passage through the birth canal and its associated physiological changes are, like quickening, implausible criteria on which to base fundamental moral distinctions.

These are complex and contentious issues. Perhaps seeking to avoid becoming embroiled in them, doctors sometimes think that unless they confront a particular medicomoral problem in their practice—for example, abortion—they do not need to bother too much about the moral arguments concerning it. But is it not obvious that any doctor who ever accepts the moral legitimacy of abortion as a bona fide medical practice—and most do—really needs to work out why he can justify abortion but not killing his adult patients? In particular, ought he not to work out what morally relevant characteristics the abortable fetus lacks that are present in his adult patients, lack of which justifies the deliberate medical killing of the fetus when there is deep moral and legal opprobrium for the deliberate medical killing of adult patients? A very similar question applies to any doctor who supports what Dr Arthur did or, more generally, who believes that newly born severely handicapped infants may in some circumstances be killed or actively "allowed to die." What morally relevant characteristics are lacking in such infants that are present in adult patients? Alternatively, what morally relevant characteristics are present in such infants that require us to treat them differently from fetuses at various stages of their development?

Handicapped neonates and handicapped adults

One sort of answer to the first question is that there is no morally relevant difference between newborn infants with serious handicaps and adults with similar handicaps and that both groups should be treated similarly. What is morally permissible treatment for handicapped newborn infants is morally permissible for similarly handicapped adults and vice versa, and what is morally impermissible for handicapped adults is morally impermissible for similarly handicapped newborn infants, and vice versa. The first thing to note is that this leaves the abortion question unanswered: if the newly born handicapped infant ought to be treated in the same way as any other patient with an equivalent handicap, how has it changed since it was an abortable handicapped fetus? Secondly, this position rules out medical management of severely diseased or handicapped newborn infants that would be unjustifiable in similarly diseased or handicapped adults or older children. Thus a doctor who held this line and believed that the prescribing of dihydrocodeine and nursing care only would be wrong for an adult or older child with Down's syndrome would also have to reject Dr Arthur's action, as the "moral prosecution" argued. (To avoid this conclusion it might be argued that in fact Dr Arthur believed in those first few days that the infant had various probably fatal and untreatable cardiac and other abnormalities in addition to Down's syndrome, as the pathologist eventually showed. I know of no reason to make such an assumption, and no evidence was given at the trial to support it.)

Standards of medical care

To avoid the conclusion that management such as Dr Arthur's of an infant with uncomplicated Down's syndrome is morally wrong it might be argued that similar management would be justifiable with an older child or adult with uncomplicated Down's syndrome. How could such a line be sustained when it would allow a doctor, when faced with a patient with uncomplicated Down's syndrome whose parents do not wish it to live, to keep the patient in hospital; withhold any medical care he would normally be given; administer large doses of dihydrocodeine, knowing its depressive effects on respiration and appetite; and feed and hydrate the patient only on demand? Surely that would not be morally acceptable in an adult or older child with uncomplicated Down's syndrome? Why not? Because it would be widely agreed by doctors and society that having Down's syndrome does not in itself justify a reduction in the standards of medical care that patients in general are owed and which are not met by this hypothetical management of "nursing care only," large doses of dihydrocodeine, and feeding and hydration only on demand.

That is not to argue that if one believes that the newly born infant with Down's syndrome should be treated like any other patient then he or she has to be treated with the most effective available medical treatment in all circumstances. Ex hypothesi the same sort of moral assessment would apply to proposed treatments for the infant as for any other patient. What treatment would the patient choose if he could deliberate about it (proxy respect for autonomy)? How much net benefit over harm can reasonably be expected for the patient (beneficence and non-maleficence)? Here the precise nature of the medical condition, the degree of handicap, the expected effects on the patient of the management proposed, and the probability of achieving for the patient a substantial net benefit over harm are crucial moral issues and will all vary according to the circumstances. Finally, would the proposed treatment be just or fair to the patient and to others, both in the burdens it imposes on all concerned and in the benefits it offers to the patient and any other beneficiaries in comparison with the resources it removes from others (justice)?

These, I have suggested, are standard moral questions that should apply to all medical care and use of medical resources, but the important thing is that they would apply no more and no less when considering the newly born infant with Down's syndrome than in any other allocation of lifesaving medical resources, if doctors owe the newly born infant with Down's syndrome the same moral obligations that they owe to all their patients.

Down's syndrome and moral rights

But perhaps they don't. One possible line of argument supporting a distinction between the moral obligations of doctors to patients with Down's syndrome and to patients in general might be that having Down's syndrome gives people fewer moral rights against doctors than they would otherwise have. Expressed in terms of doctors' duties, the claim would be that if a patient has Down's syndrome doctors have less stringent moral obligations towards him or her than they would normally have. But how could such a claim be justified? Without a rationale it is no more convincing than a similar claim about patients with Gilbert's syndrome or those who happen to have blue eyes. Perhaps the justification offered would be that Down's syndrome results in such a low quality of life compared with normal human flourishing that doctors are not morally obliged to treat patients with Down's syndrome? This is an argument that the right to life organisations and many others find particularly objectionable—rightly so.

Its implications are that people with Down's syndrome of any age and development, and any degree of handicap, are morally second class and can be "allowed to die" when those in the first class would be kept alive. Moreover, it implies that the same sort of moral discrimination is justified against anyone else with a similar quality of life to that of the least impaired person with Down's syndrome. Given the varying degrees of quality of life and the wide range of flourishing that older children and adults with Down's syndrome manifest, the argument that any person with Down's syndrome may be denied lifesaving medical care, let alone that such people may be actively "allowed to die," is clearly morally unacceptable. But why is it morally unacceptable? The answer is surely that there is something about the nature of older children and adults with Down's syndrome that makes us recognise a moral obligation to

treat them as we treat each other. But what is different about them
(*a*) compared with newborn infants with Down's syndrome, if we
believe that we can treat the latter in lifethreatening ways that we
find morally unacceptable in relation to other patients, including
older patients with Down's syndrome; and (*b*) compared with
embryos and fetuses with Down's syndrome, if we believe that we
may justifiably kill (abort) these?

What is a person?

One radical and contentious answer is that fetuses and newly born
humans, whether they have Down's syndrome or not, are not
people, whereas older children and adults, including those with
Down's syndrome, are. According to this line of argument the
"right to life" is a right of people or persons; the moral obligation not
to kill others is a duty not to kill other people or persons. What is
meant by "a person" and "people" in this context is inadequately
worked out and a subject of vigorous philosophical debate. One line
of argument is that a necessary condition for being a person, and
thus for being owed the moral respect due to persons, including an
intrinsic (though prima facie) moral right not to be intentionally
killed by others, is awareness of oneself or self consciousness. (This
line of argument stems from a discussion about the nature of persons
by the physician-philosopher John Locke.[4]) It seems plausible that
the morally special attributes that distinguish people from animals
and other entities to which we do not accord an intrinsic right to life
require a capacity for self consciousness. According to this argument self consciousness is not morally important in itself but is a
necessary condition of all the remarkable and distinguishing
characteristics that endow people with special moral importance
and thus special moral rights. This argument supposes that all
newborn infants, like all fetuses, are not self conscious and therefore
cannot be people and therefore do not have an intrinsic moral right
to life. Clearly part of the argument rests on empirical claims and
requires appropriate empirical support, but there seems little doubt
that newly fertilised ova are not self conscious and equally little
doubt that adults are, therefore somewhere along the developmental
line, perhaps gradually rather than suddenly, self consciousness
must develop.

The right to life and newborn infants

Of course, even if this argument were accepted it does not imply that fetuses and babies should not in most cases be carefully protected. There are several justifications for such protection other than an intrinsic right to life. The first is that the development from newly fertilised ovum to self conscious human being is gradual, and there are plausible consequentialist reasons for reflecting such development by according gradually increasing moral protection to the developing embryo, fetus, and newly born infant. Secondly, in most cases mothers, fathers, families, and societies put enormous value on newly born babies—much greater value than, in our society, they typically put on the embryo and fetus—and thus there are important consequentialist reasons for reflecting this distinction in our social institutions. Thirdly, in most cases great personal and social anguish and disruption would result if newly born babies were not given very careful protection, especially by doctors.

None the less, if it is true that newly born infants have not yet developed into people and therefore do not yet have the full moral rights of people, including the "right to life," then it becomes justifiable for societies to determine that in certain circumstances the protection that should normally be extended to newly born infants may be withdrawn. In cases where an intrinsic right to life did not exist to function as a moral "trump card" such circumstances would be determined by considerations of overall harm and benefit, which took into account both the moral repugnance normally evinced at infanticide and also the harm to families and society of keeping alive unwanted severely handicapped infants. Given the great social disagreement over these issues it would, of course, be intolerable—even in merely consequentialist terms—to impose any such withdrawal of protection or "allowing to die." If the parents of severely handicapped newborn infants want them to be medically sustained then their wishes should if possible be respected—but if, having considered the matter, the parents want the infant to be painlessly "allowed to die" then according to this argument their wishes too can legitimately be respected.

The question of acts and omissions

Many doctors would support active "allowing to die" of the sort carried out by Dr Arthur but would reject any active killing of such infants. I believe I have shown that it is difficult to justify even active "allowing to die" unless it is also agreed that severely handicapped newborn infants are not owed the same moral duties, especially the duty to preserve their lives, that doctors owe to their patients in general. I have also argued previously, however, against the customary medical assumption that the distinction between acts and omissions can justify a moral distinction between withdrawal of medical treatment and active killing. A moral question has to be answered first—namely, which medical acts and omissions to act are morally justifiable and which are not? Knowingly causing conditions in which an infant is likely to die when it is otherwise unlikely to do so, and where there is no intention of benefiting the infant by doing so, is normally regarded as morally culpable, as murder or manslaughter. The father who killed baby Brown, also an infant with Down's syndrome, was jailed for manslaughter. What are the morally important differences between what he did and what Dr Arthur did?[5][6] There is no reason to suppose that the verdict on baby Brown's father would have been ameliorated had his baby died because the father gave dihydrocodeine, fed and hydrated it only on demand, and then did not obtain medical care when it became ill. Such treatment could only be justified if (a) the newborn infant, like the fetus, does not have an intrinsic right to life and (b) there is sufficient justification in terms of overall benefit over harm (in this context restriction of such treatments to doctors and parents acting together may help to minimise the harm).

A radical challenge

Here, then, is a radical challenge to those who would support Dr Arthur's action. If they believe that they owe the same duty to respect the lives of newborn infants with Down's syndrome as they owe to all their other patients how do they justify their support of actions that they would almost certainly reject in older patients with Down's syndrome? (And if they also defend abortion—for example, of fetuses with Down's syndrome—how do they justify their different attitudes to the fetus and to the newborn infant?) If, on the other hand, they believe that they do not owe the same duty to newborn infants with Down's syndrome that they owe to their other patients, how do they justify this position without falling into the trap of denying all patients with Down's syndrome the moral protection they afford to their patients in general? I believe that the issue turns on the question of personhood and that it is because the newly born infant is not a person that it is justifiable in cases of severe handicap to "allow it to die" in the way Dr Arthur allowed baby Pearson to die. But while there may be some social benefits in distinguishing between actively "allowing to die" and painlessly killing such infants, there is, I believe, no other moral difference, and doctors who accept such "allowing to die" of severely handicapped newborn infants should not deceive themselves into believing that there is such a difference. Those who do not accept these radical claims yet wish to support action like Dr Arthur's need to cudgel their brains for a rationale, one that is consistent with their attitudes to abortion, the "morning after pill," embryo research, and the treatment of newborn infants with spina bifida or anencephaly, of patients with severe dementia, of patients in persistent vegetative state, and of those with "brain stem death." Such are the widespread ramifications of questions about the scope of our moral obligations to human beings at different stages of their lives.

References

1 Beauchamp TL, Childress JF. *Principles of biomedical ethics*. 2nd ed. New York, Oxford: Oxford University Press, 1983.
2 Jonsen AR, Siegler M, Winslade WJ. *Clinical ethics*. London: Baillière Tindall, 1982.
3 Brody H. *Ethical decisions in medicine*. 2nd ed. Boston: Little Brown, 1981.
4 Locke J. *Essay concerning human understanding*. Book 2: chapter 27, section 9. London, 1690.
5 Davis JA. The "baby Brown" case and the Dr Arthur verdict. *J Med Ethics* 1985;11:159.
6 Kennedy I. Response to professor Davis. *J Med Ethics* 1985;11:159-60.

Index